Schools Council History 13–16 Project

MEDICINE THROUGH TIME

A study in development

BOOK ONE

Early man and medicine

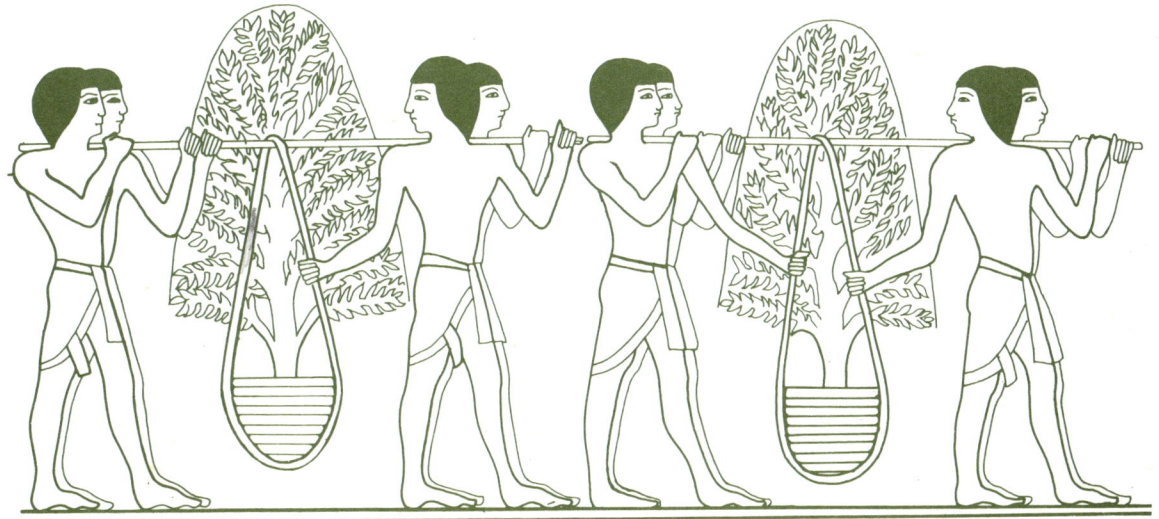

HOLMES MCDOUGALL EDINBURGH

Schools Council History 13–16 Project

This project was set up in 1972 at the University of Leeds and continued there for five years with a Schools Council grant of £126 000.

Its main aim was to suggest suitable objectives for history teachers, and to promote the use of appropriate materials and ideas for their realisation. This involved a reconsideration of the nature of history and its relevance in secondary schools; the design of a syllabus framework which shows the uses that history may have in the education of adolescents; and the setting-up of experimental O Level and CSE examinations.

Project Team

David Sylvester (Director to 1975)
Tony Boddington (Director from 1975)
Gwenifer Griffiths (1975–1976)
William Harrison (1972–1975)
John Mann (1974–1975)
Aileen Plummer (from 1972)
Denis Shemilt (Evaluator, from 1974)
Peter Wenham (to 1974)

Design and illustration by Edward Burrill

Holmes McDougall
Allander House
137–141 Leith Walk
Edinburgh EH6 8NS

ISBN 0 7157 1583–6

Printed by Holmes McDougall   Edinburgh

Contents

1. Medicine and disease in prehistoric times

Learn about trephining [handwritten note]

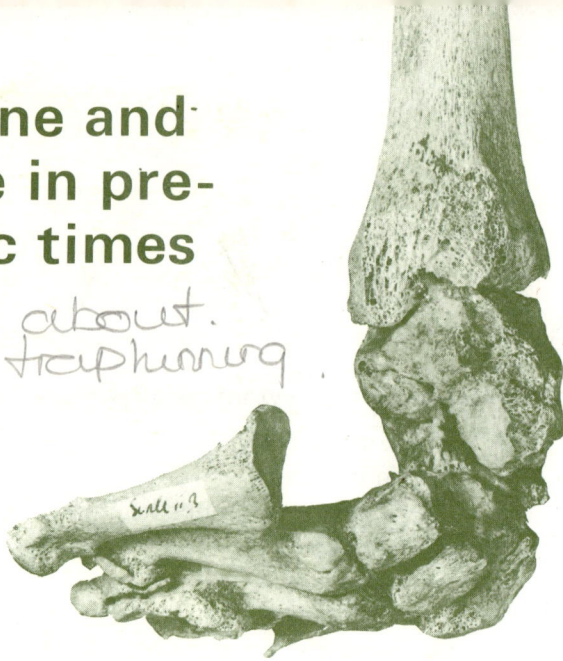

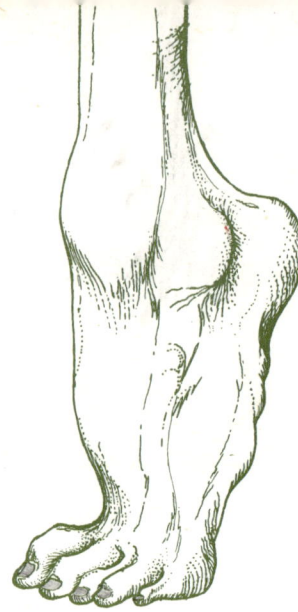

A prehistoric case of clubfoot

The clubfoot of Siptah, an Egyptian pharaoh (drawn from a photograph of his mummified body)

Evidence from prehistoric times

We know from the evidence of bones and skeletons that disease and sickness were present in prehistoric times around seventeen thousand years ago. We do not know, however, exactly how people at this time dealt with the problem of disease because they left us no written record of their beliefs and practices. We do not know how much they knew about the structure and workings of the human body. We cannot be sure how they treated sickness or what they believed to be its causes.

As you can see, a few pieces of evidence have survived and these may be able to tell us something about medicine in prehistoric times. Yet this evidence is not enough. It tells us a little but it can be interpreted in different ways and so we need to look for other clues.

Unfortunately at present we have little direct evidence about prehistoric medicine. But it may be possible to find *some* clues by studying people whose way of life, in certain aspects, resembled that of prehistoric men and women until recent times. One such group of people is the Australian Aborigines. Obviously, we must *not* assume that their beliefs and culture were exactly the same as those of prehistoric people. However, by studying Aboriginal ideas about medicine and disease we may perhaps be able to interpret some of the evidence relating to disease and its treament in prehistoric times.

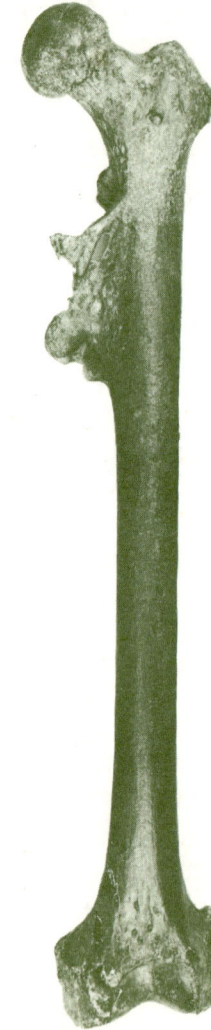

The femur (a leg bone) of a prehistoric man showing a bony outgrowth

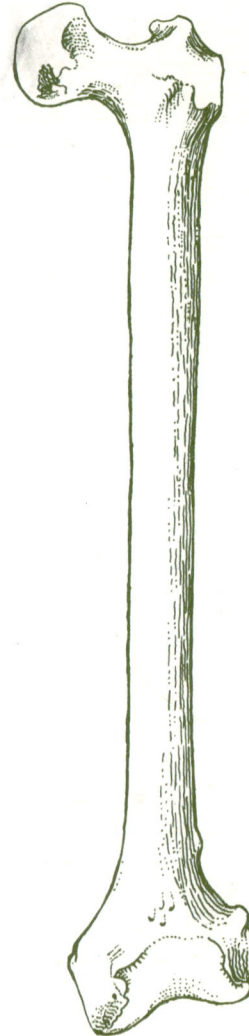

A normal femur for comparison

A cave painting from southern France

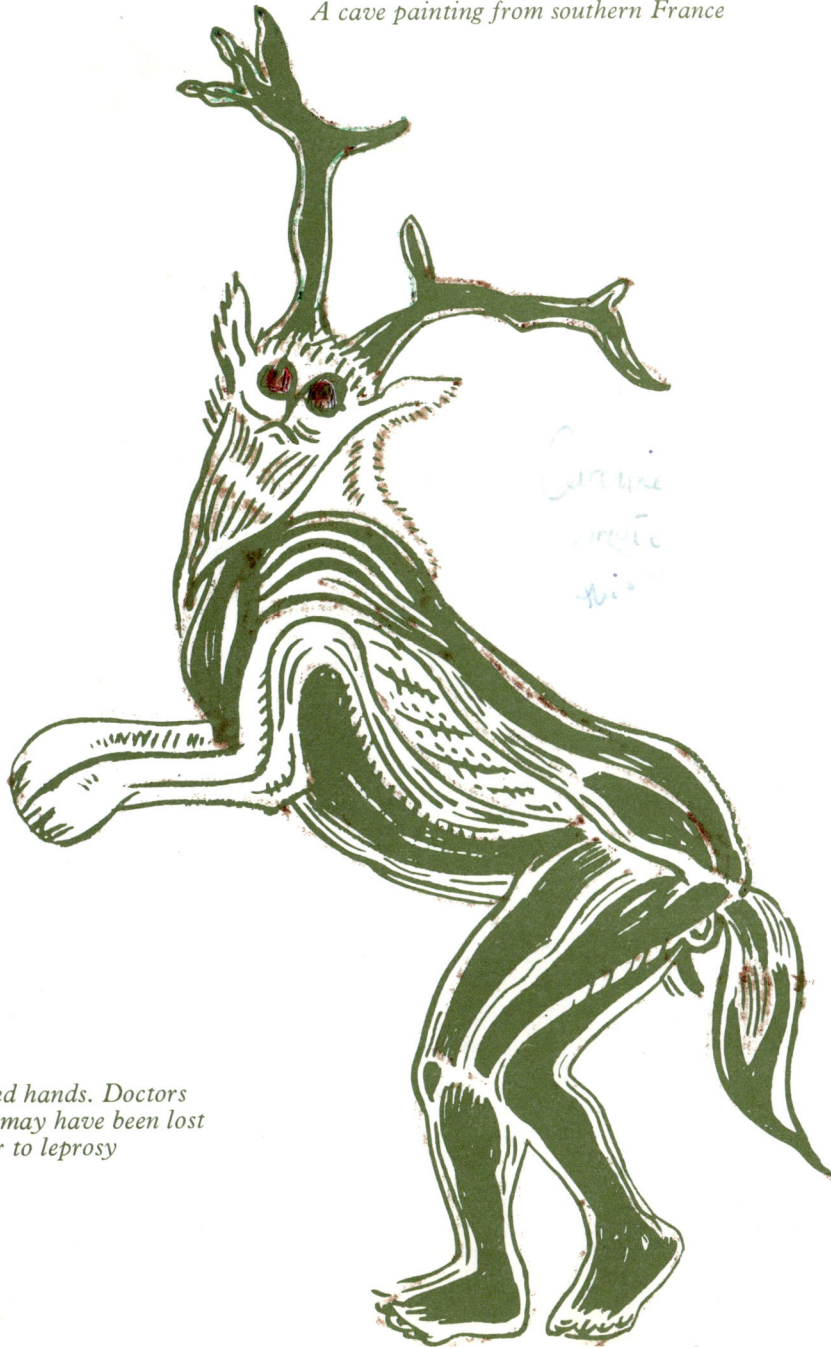

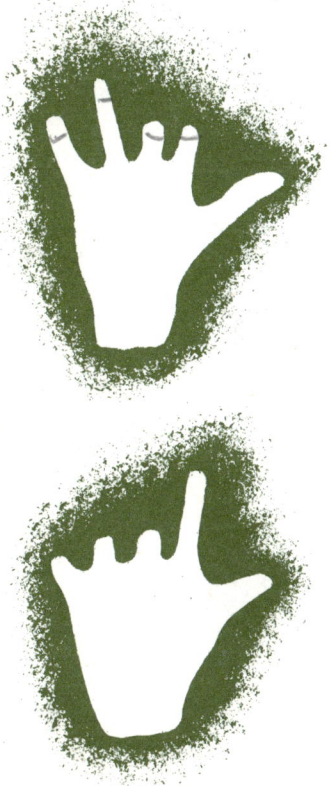

Prehistoric skull : notice the circular holes which have been made in the skull. Flint scrapers were probably used to perform this kind of surgical operation which is known as trephinning. Hundreds of such skulls have been found all over the world. Many of them show that the bone round the hole has started to grow again proving that the man lived after the operation. Few of the skulls showed any injuries indicating that this was not an operation designed to repair a fractured skull

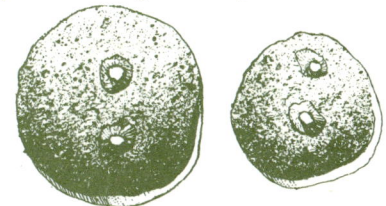

Stone age imprints of mutilated hands. Doctors think that parts of the fingers may have been lost due to diseased blood vessels or to leprosy

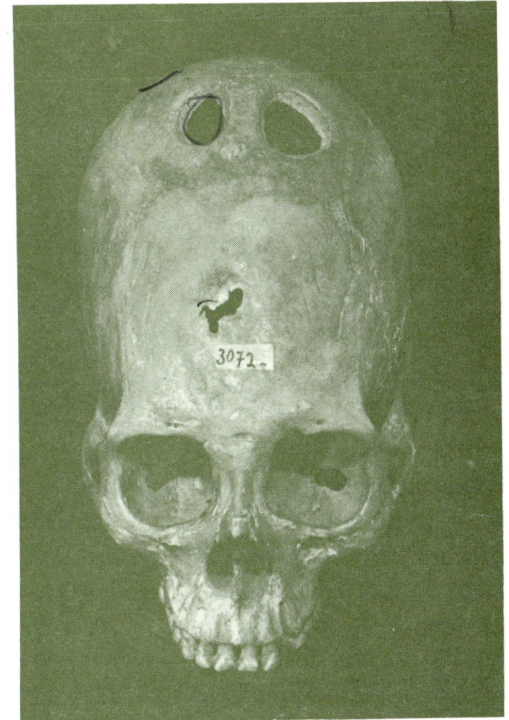

Two pieces of bone from the circular holes in a trephinned skull. Small holes have been drilled in the middle suggesting that they may have been threaded with a leather thong and worn around the neck

The Australian Aborigines

The Aborigines were the first inhabitants of Australia. Until recent times they were a Stone Age people in the sense that all their weapons and tools were made of stone or wood.

Because Australia had no plants which could be cultivated and no animals which could be domesticated (apart from dogs), the Aborigines had to live by hunting kangaroos, wallabies and other animals, by fishing and by gathering roots, grubs, and berries. Large areas of Australia have little rain and there is much desert and semi-desert land. Many Aborigines in central Australia often had to wander over their tribal lands in search of water or water-giving plants.

Such a nomadic life meant that the Aborigines had no need of permanent homes and so when necessary they made themselves temporary shelters of tree-bark. Although they had over six hundred spoken languages, the Aborigines had no written language. Many, however, were skilful artists and produced beautiful drawings of humans and animals on sheets of bark or on cave walls.

As many of their drawings show, the Aborigines were close and accurate observers of the world around them. Indeed, their survival depended on their skill at observing and tracking animals and finding roots, berries and—most important—water. A detailed knowledge of certain aspects of the natural world was especially important to the tribes which lived in the more hostile environment of central Australia.

At the same time, the Aborigines appear to have had no scientific explanations for certain natural phenomena such as the wind, the rain or the seasons. It also seems likely that before any contact with Europeans the Aborigines did not know the scientific facts about human conception and reproduction.

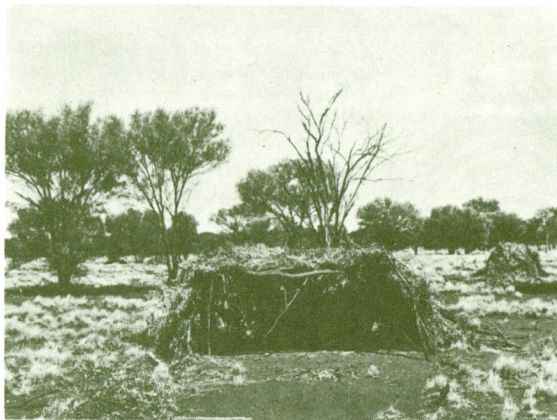

An Aboriginal shelter

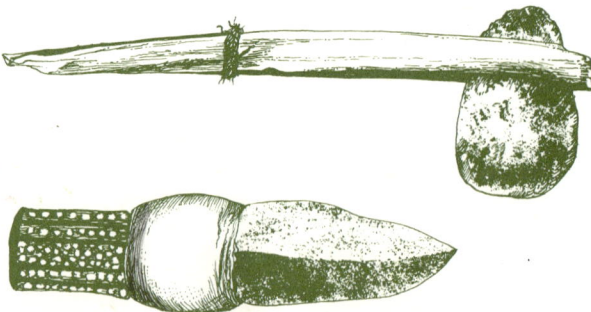

Stone axe and knife

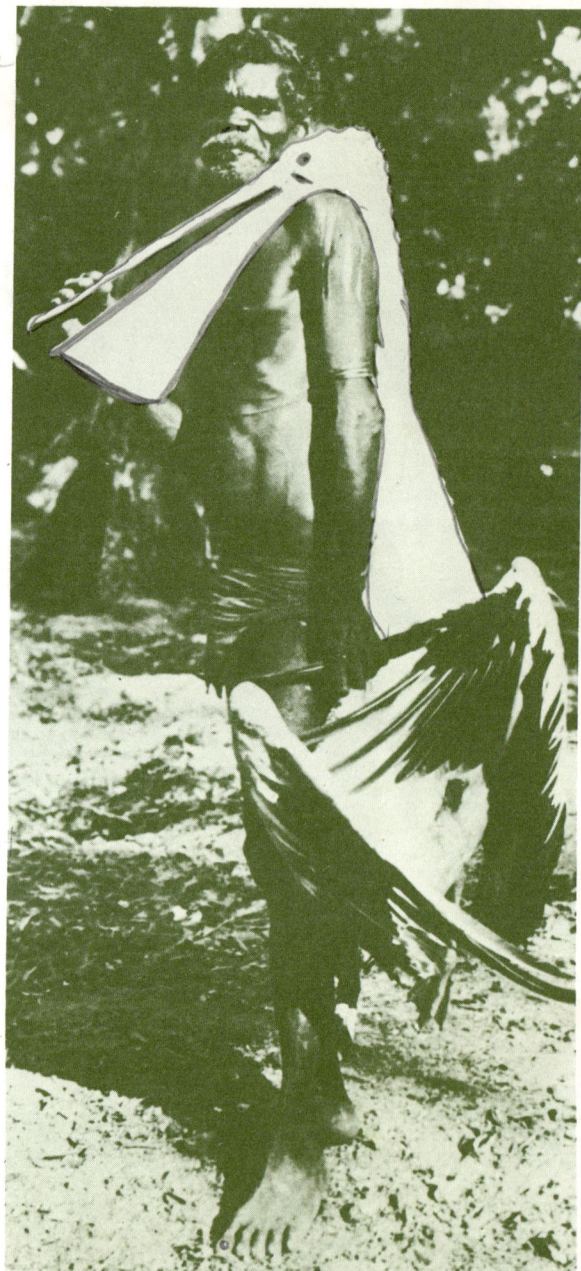

An Aborigine with a pelican

6

The spirit world of the Aborigines

The Aborigines developed their own myths and legends which provided explanations for the origin of life and for the world of nature. The natural world, they believed, was full of spirits. These spirits were present in all things and so were everywhere.

According to Aboriginal legend, long ago in an age called 'The Dreamtime' the first animals, plants, rivers, mountains and human beings, were created by a group of spirits whom the Aborigines called their spirit ancestors. These spirit ancestors were huge and wonderful creatures. Some were human, some animal, and some were part-human and part-animal. There were creatures such as the Rainbow Serpent, the Emu Man, the Fish Ancestor and the Mosquito Man.

During their time on earth, the spirit ancestors created all things. The Kangaroo Man made a sacred pole and then turned it into a gum tree. When the Sun Man stole another man's wife, the husband became angry. He stabbed his wife in the stomach, water poured out and a lake was formed. The Rainbow Serpent made the rivers as he slid along. Once their work was done, the time came for the spirit ancestors to go. Some disappeared into the ground leaving waterholes and piles of rock to mark the spot. Others turned into trees or became rock paintings.

When they went, however, the ancestors left spirit children in the place from which they disappeared. These spirit children were to remain forever in that place waiting for a chance to be reborn as a new plant, animal or human being.

The spirit children gave rise to all the continuing human, plant and animal life around the Aborigines. For example, if an Aborigine woman chanced to walk near the disappearing place of the Emu Man, a spirit child left by the Emu Man could enter her body and grow into a human baby. Another spirit could enter the emu bird and become an emu chick. Because of this, all humans and birds born of the Emu Man's spirits were thought to be spirit brothers. All men and women had a spirit brother in nature— be it plant or animal.

As long as an Aborigine's spirit stayed within his or her body that person would be well and happy. But people had to beware in case the spirit escaped through an open mouth during sleep. On death all spirits returned to the disappearing place of their ancestor and waited there to be reborn.

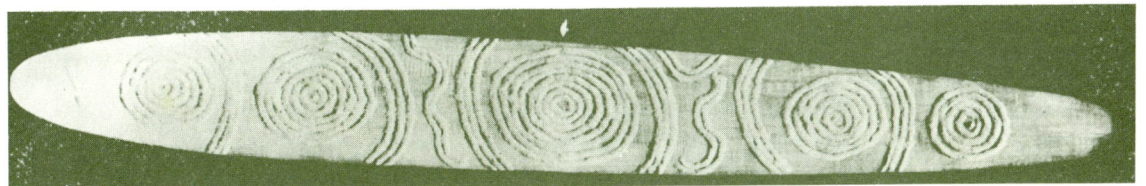

A sacred churinga stone : the carved designs are meant to represent the places sacred to one of the spirit ancestors, such as water holes and paths

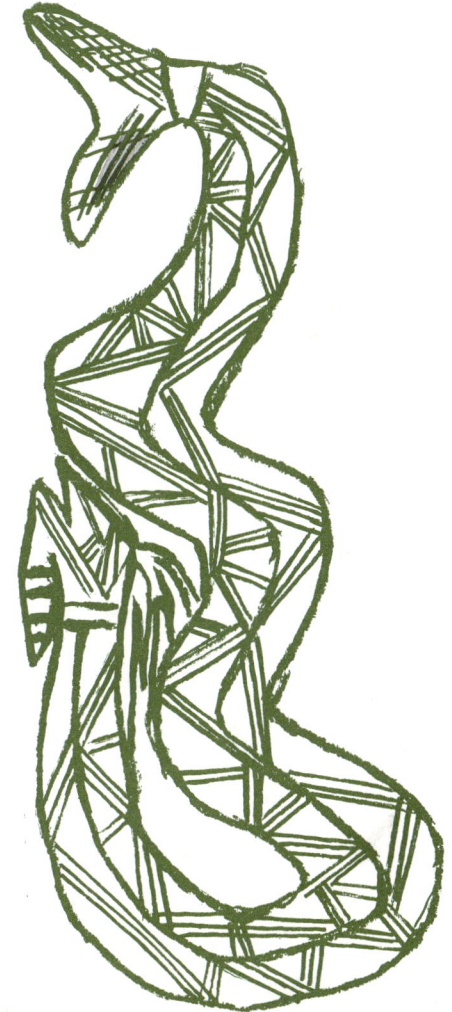

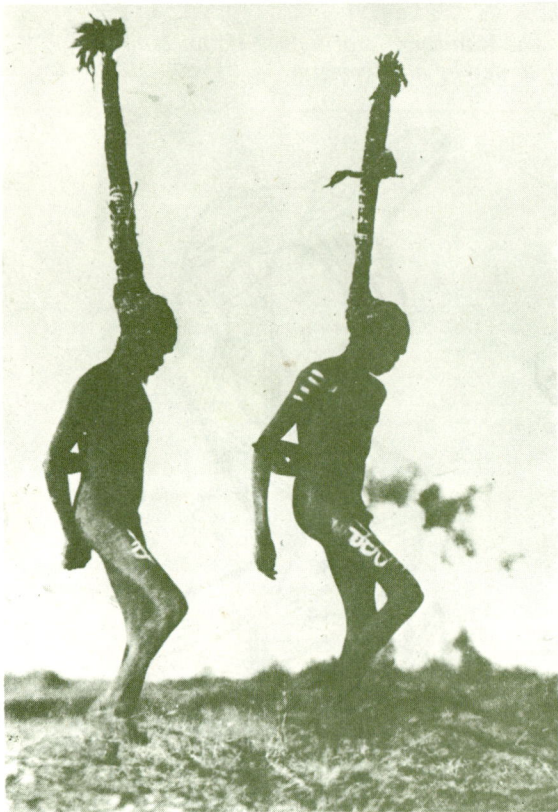

Aborigine Emu dancers

According to Aborigine legend, the spirit ancestors created landscape features such as rocks and water holes

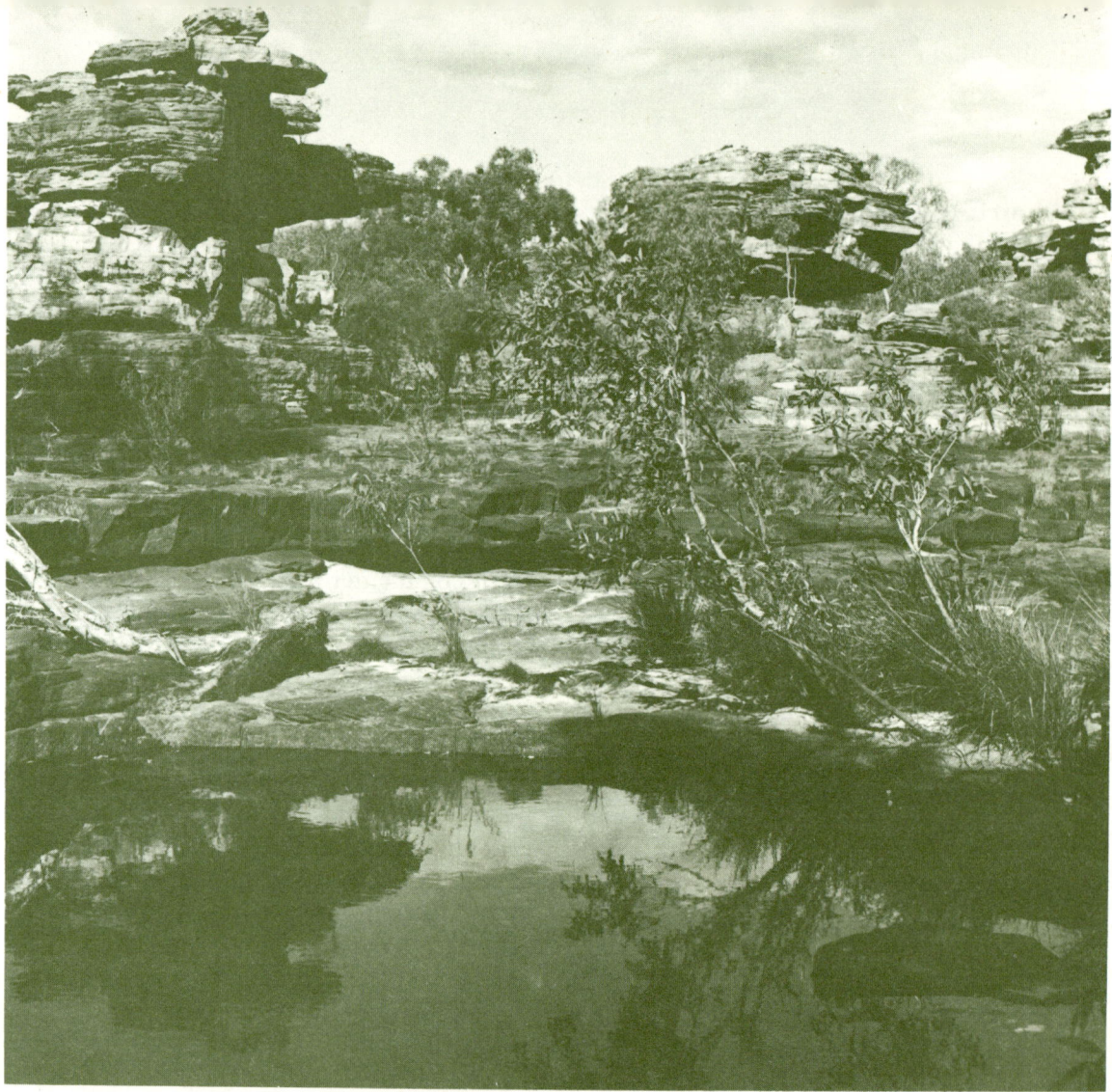

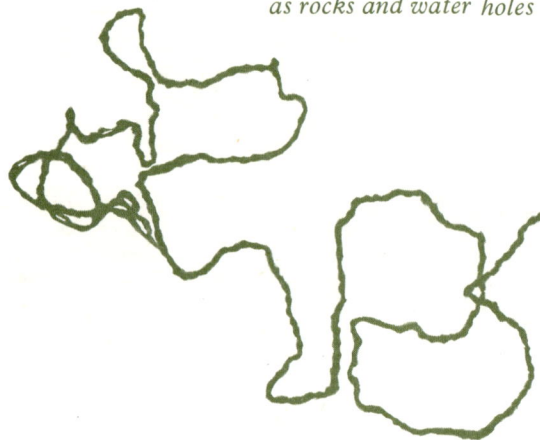

A bullroarer : a wooden sacred object which when whirled in the air makes a droning noise. Women and children believe that the noise made by the bullroarer is the voice of a spirit ancestor

Aboriginal medicine

The Aborigines, then, developed their own explanations for the origin of life and certain natural phenomena. These were different from the explanations that we would use. They were, however, just as complex and they did help the Aborigines to make sense of the world around them. The Aborigines also developed their own explanations for the cause of disease and their own methods of treatment, both of which were closely connected with their knowledge and understanding of the natural world.

There were two aspects of Aboriginal medicine. One of them was concerned with the treatment of everyday ailments and injuries, most of which had an obvious cause. For such complaints the Aborigines had a wide range of simple but effective remedies. These remedies were based on experience and rational common sense.

By a process of observation, trial and error, and perhaps even instinct, the Aborigines had discovered the value of plants and other medicinal substances in the treatment of certain ailments. They also knew that heat helped to relieve pain and swelling, and had learned how to deal with certain fractures. Here are some of the remedies they used: *open cuts* were covered with a pad of mud, clay, or animal fat, or closed up with an eaglehawk feather and bound with layers of paper bark and kangaroo skin, *burns* were smeared with animal fat or sap from trees, *dysentery* was treated by chewing young shoots or an orchid bulb, *broken arms* were encased in mud and clay, *rheumatic pains, fevers and swellings* were were treated with steam from a pit of damped green grass laid on burning bark.

The second aspect of Aboriginal medicine was concerned with the treatment of illnesses which had no obvious cause, or which did

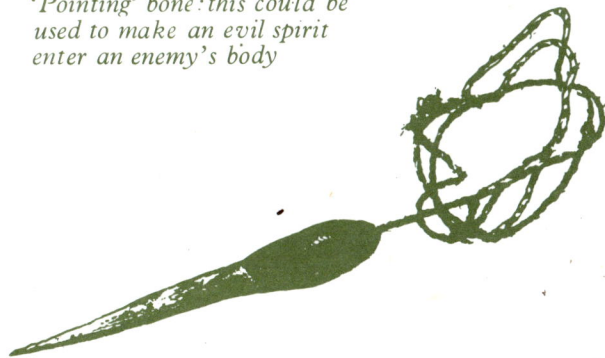

'Pointing' bone: this could be used to make an evil spirit enter an enemy's body

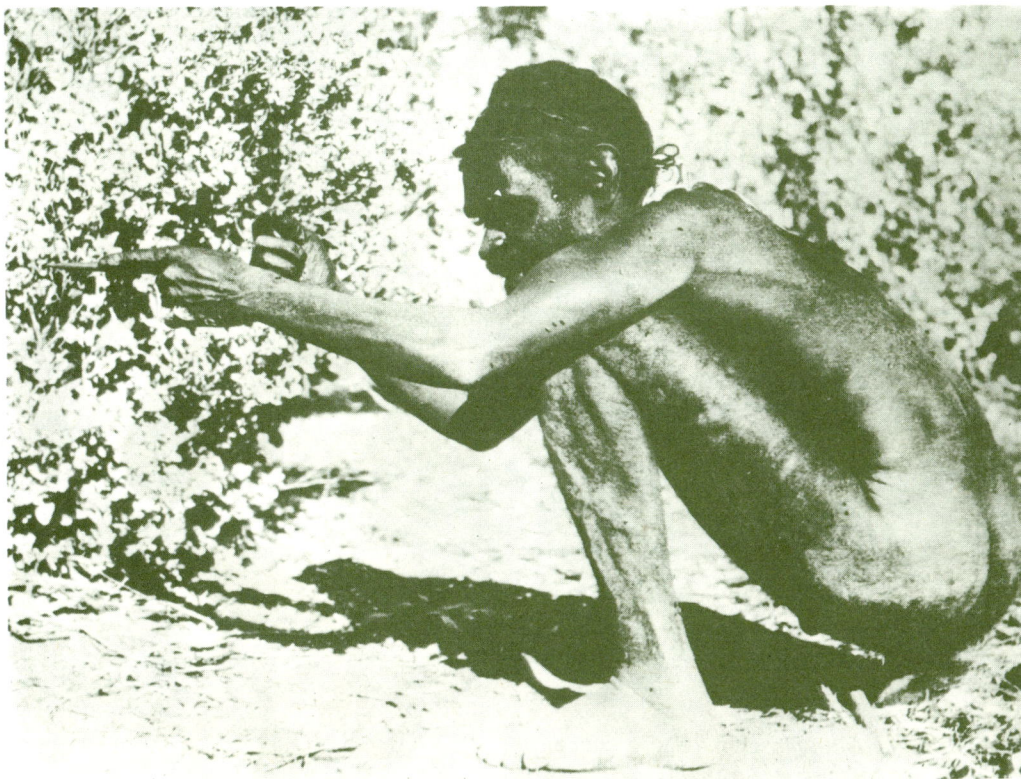

A Medicine Man in the Northern Territory shows how the magic bone is 'pointed' at a victim while he is 'singing'

not respond to common-sense remedies. The Aborigines believed that these ailments were connected with spirits and could be caused in two ways: either an evil spirit could enter their bodies and so cause disease, or their own spirits could be enticed away.

Some tribes believed that there were evil spirits which lived in holes in gum trees. At night these spirits wandered around and if they entered the bodies of sleeping people they could cause sickness or death.

An enemy could make an evil spirit enter a person's body by chanting (or, as the Aborigines would say, by 'singing') and pointing a bone in his or her direction. These 'pointing bones' could also be used to catch a spirit and pull it from the body and so cause sickness or death. The bone was pointed towards a victim and the chants were sung. The victim's spirit left the body and was caught on some gum at the end of the bone. The spirit was then absorbed into the bone. Finally the bone was wrapped in emu feathers and buried. This signalled the person's doom unless treatment was sought.

The Medicine Man

Serious illnesses which were thought to be caused by evil spirits were usually treated by the Medicine Man. These men were believed to have power over evil spirits. They carried quartz crystals which were considered to be the source of their powers. Some tribes believed that the Medicine Man was given his magical powers by the ancestors.

When called to a sick person, the Medicine Man first had to question every member of the family carefully to diagnose the cause of the illness. Was there an enemy who might have pointed the bone? Had the person felt the spirit leave?

To cure the illness the Medicine Man then had to 'extract' the evil spirit from his patient's body or find and replace the patient's own spirit. If 'extraction' was called for, the Medicine Man would first sing the sick man or woman into a trance, massaging the sore part of the body and sucking it vigorously for some time. Eventually by sleight of hand he would produce a quartz crystal in which the evil spirit was believed to be hiding.

If the patient's spirit had been stolen, the Medicine Man had to find the 'pointing bone' which had been used to trap the spirit. He then had to throw the 'pointing bone' into water and set the captive spirit free.

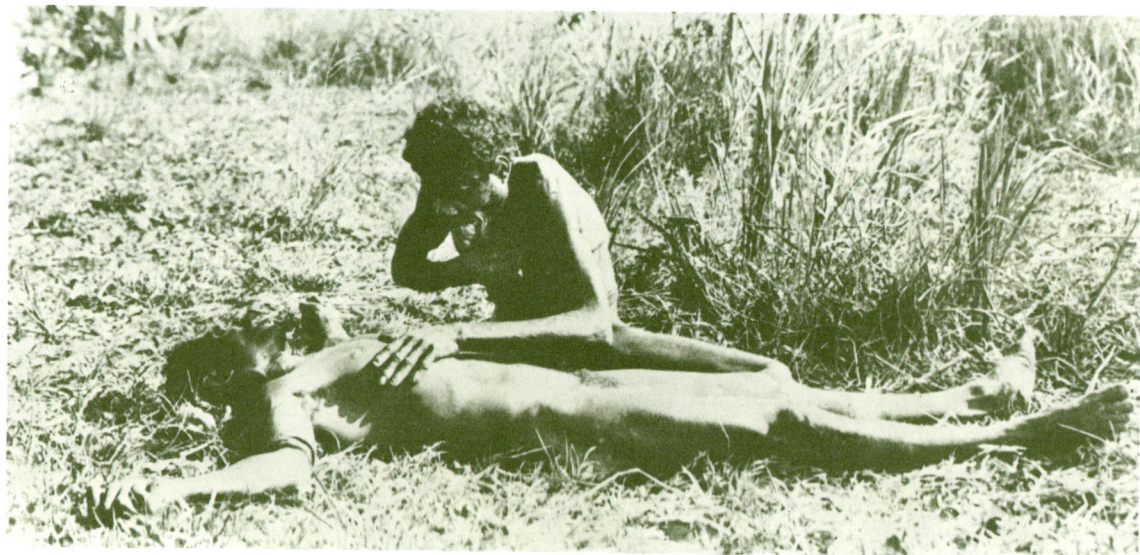

A Medicine Man massaging a sick man with sweat from his own armpits

Health and hygiene

The Aborigines also believed that they could prevent disease by wearing charms to ward off evil spirits. Some of these charms were made from parts of a human body or the seeds of a plant.

It is unlikely that the Aborigines had any scientific understanding of the connection between hygiene and the prevention of disease. In certain ways, however, their beliefs and way of life did help to protect their health. Their natural environment contained very few of the many organisms which can cause infectious disease. Before their contact with Europeans, the Aborigines did not wear clothes, and this also helped to protect them from disease.

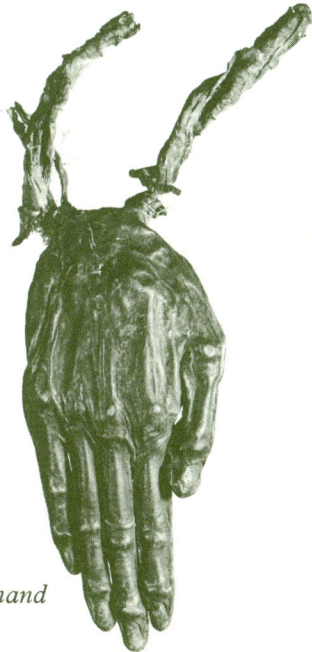

A charm made from a human hand

Because Aborigines moved from place to place so frequently there was little danger to their health from poor sanitation. Some tribes were careful to bury their excrement and cast-off hair and nails. We do not know exactly why they did this. Some anthropologists believe that the Aborigines did not want any part of their body to fall into the hands of an enemy, because it could then be used to work evil magic against them. But this practice could have been a simple hygiene precaution.

Primitive people and medicine

These then, were some of the beliefs and practices of one group of primitive people until recent times. It is interesting to note how the magical and rational beliefs of the Aborigines combined to provide them with a medical lore which was more than adequate for their way of life. It also seems likely that their lack of scientific medical knowledge was no great disadvantage as long as the Aborigines were able to avoid the diseases (especially infectious diseases) imported by Europeans.

But can this information tell us anything at all about medicine in prehistoric times? We cannot make direct comparisons, but knowledge of Aboriginal medicine may help us to understand some of the *evidence* left by prehistoric peoples. Look carefully at this evidence again and see if you think our knowledge of Aboriginal medicine can provide any clues to its interpretation.

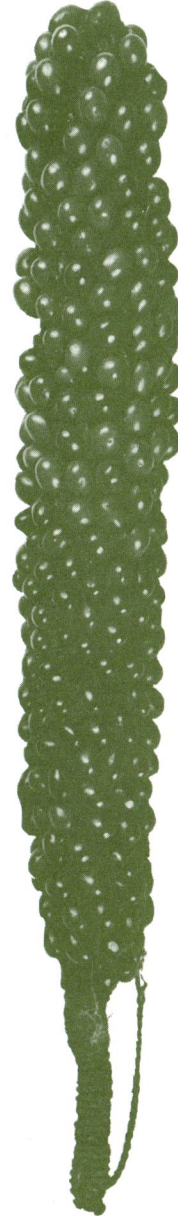

2. Drugs and doctors: a study of medicine in Ancient Egypt

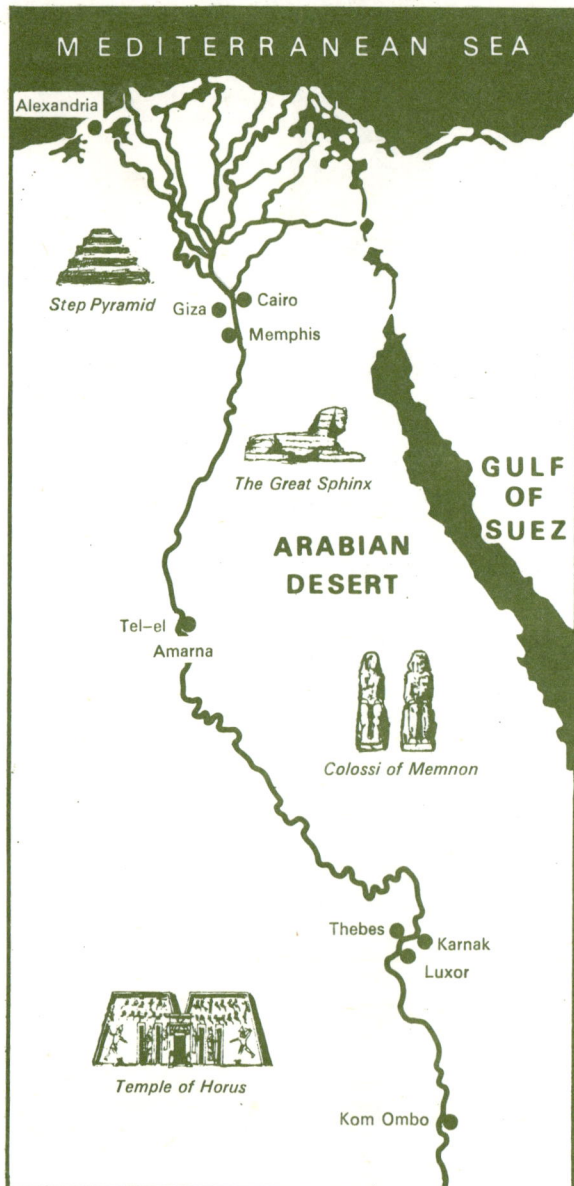

Map showing Egypt in the time of the Pharaohs

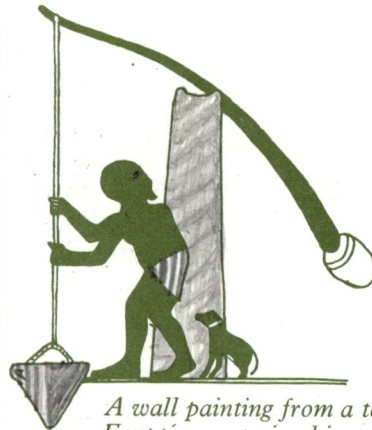

A wall painting from a tomb showing an Egyptian watering his garden with a shaduf

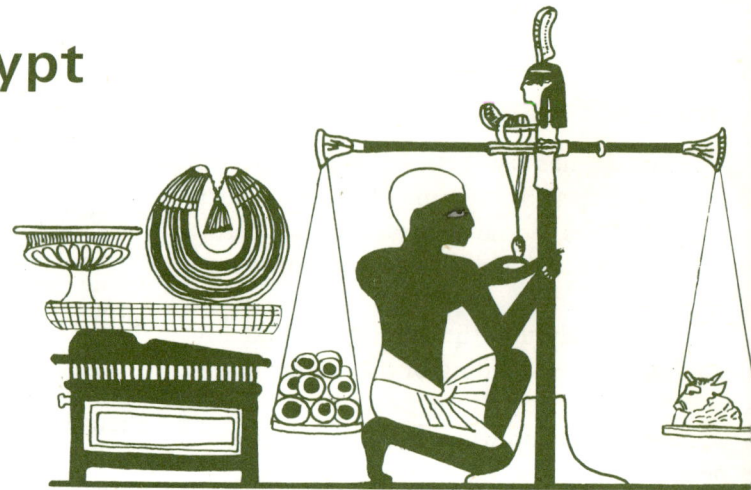

Wall painting from a tomb showing a scribe weighing out gold using a bronze bull's head weight

The Egyptians

By 3000 B.C. Egyptian civilisation was developing in the valley of the River Nile. The soil in the valley was fertile and was watered each year by the flood waters of the Nile. There were cattle which could be domesticated and grains which could be cultivated. The Egyptians, the people of the Nile valley, were therefore able to make a living by farming instead of hunting. They were able to settle in one place instead of wandering in search of food. They also learned to work together to build dams and irrigation channels which would conserve the flood waters of the Nile so that they could be used to water the fields.

Leaders were needed to organise the people in this work and in time the Pharaohs emerged as the kingly and priestly rulers of Egypt. There was now a settled system of government with cities and temples and an army. The skill of writing developed, at first using clay tablets and later papyrus. Records could now be kept, orders could be issued and history written. Methods of calculating were invented so that taxes could be computed, land surveyed, weights and distances measured and time recorded.

The fact that each man no longer had to spend all his time in search of food and

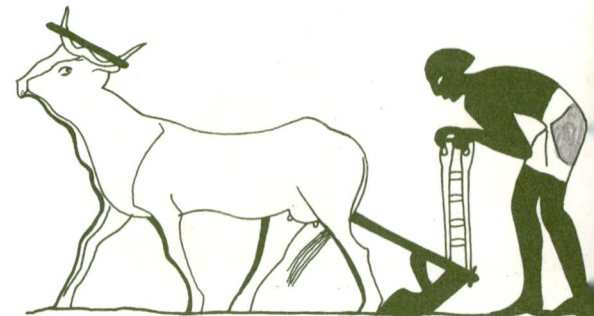

Wall painting from a tomb showing an Egyptian farmer guiding his plough

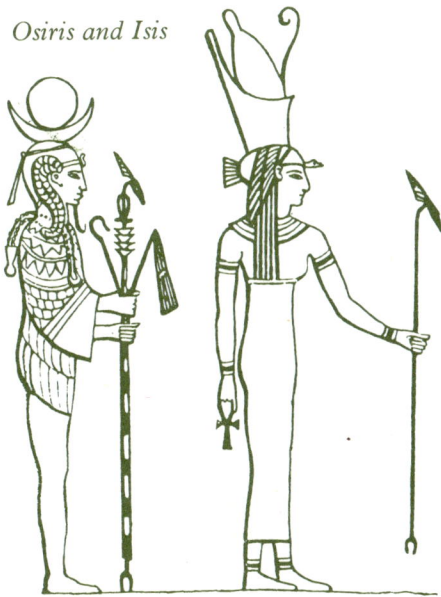

Osiris and Isis

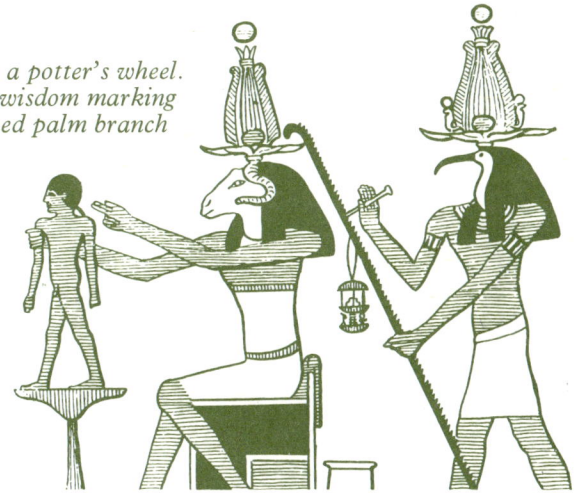

The god Khum making a man at a potter's wheel. Behind stands Thoth, the god of wisdom marking the man's years of life on a notched palm branch (from a wall painting)

shelter was very important. Some men were now free to consider other things such as the method of building pyramids or of channelling water from the river to the fields. The Egyptians not only had the time to think about these problems; because of the development of writing and calculating they also had the means to work out solutions and to record their answers. People were free to observe and study the world around them more closely and so learn more about it.

But although the Egyptians discovered much about the world, there were still many things for which they had no natural explanation. With the aid of the calendar and of 'nilometers', the Egyptians were able to predict when the Nile would flood and how far the water would rise. They had learned how to channel the flood waters, but they did not know the exact source of the Nile or *why* it flooded each year. The Egyptians also knew that every year, after

the floods, the land became fertile. Crops grew well and were ripened by the sun— but how and why did they grow and what was the sun?

The Egyptians believed that such happenings, caused by something beyond their senses, were connected with spiritual beings. They had many gods, often depicted as part-animal and part-human. Like their more primitive ancestors, the Egyptians believed that the gods had created the world and that nothing in it happened without their approval or their command.

In early times, the Egyptians had devised many myths and legends which helped to explain certain natural phenomena. They believed that there were waters under the earth which swelled up each year from subterranean caverns and caused the Nile to flood. According to legend, it was the god Osiris and his wife Isis who caused the crops to grow each year after the flood. The myth of Osiris and Isis described how Osiris was killed by Seth his wicked brother. Seth then scattered the pieces of Osiris' body all over Egypt. Isis travelled throughout the land to find and collect the pieces of her husband's

body. Eventually she was able to bring Osiris back to life and he then became god of the underworld. Each year, however, just as Osiris had died and then been reborn, so the plants too began to grow once more.

In Egyptian legend, the sun was also a god, Re. Each day he travelled across the sky in a boat, often fighting (but always defeating) Apophis, the cloud god. In the redness of sunset Re would step from his day boat to his night boat to be towed through the night on the waters which flowed under the world. At dawn he would step back into the day boat and begin his journey across the sky again.

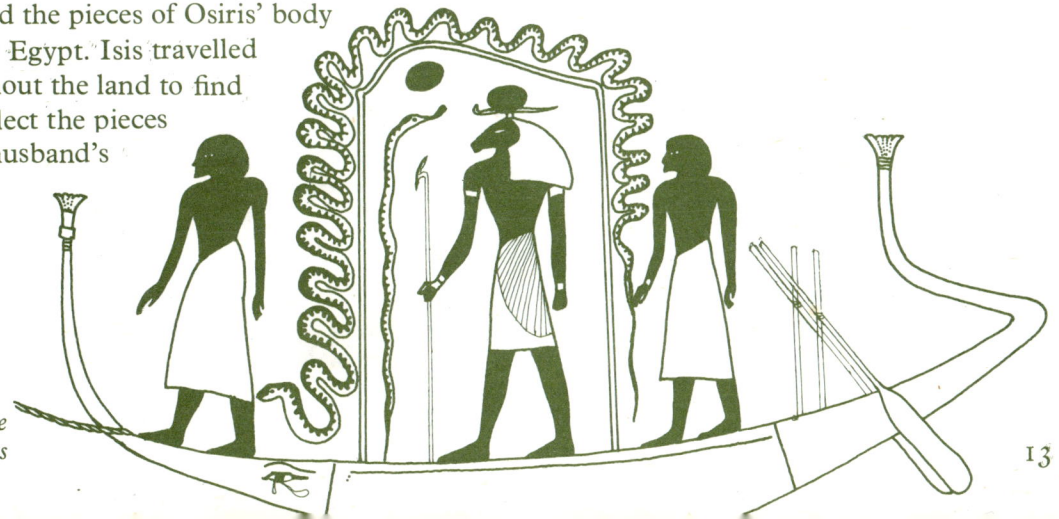

Wall painting showing Re, the sun-god, being towed on the waters under the earth during the night hours

Egyptian medicine

The first doctors

Egyptian beliefs about disease and health were closely connected with attitudes to life in general. Egyptian medicine included a mixture of old and new ideas; supernatural explanations and magical remedies were mingled with a great deal of practical common sense and a willingness to inquire and investigate.

In Ancient Egypt the treatment of sickness was no longer carried out only by magicians and medicine men. There were also physicians or doctors, as the following piece of evidence shows:

An Egyptian love poem (written about 1500 B.C.)
It is seven days from yesterday
since I saw my love,
And sickness has crept over me,
My limbs have become heavy,
I cannot feel my own body.
If the master-physicians come
to me
I gain no comfort from their
remedies.
And the priest-magicians have
no cures,
My sickness is not diagnosed.
My love is better by far for
me than any remedies.
She is more important than all
the books of medicine.

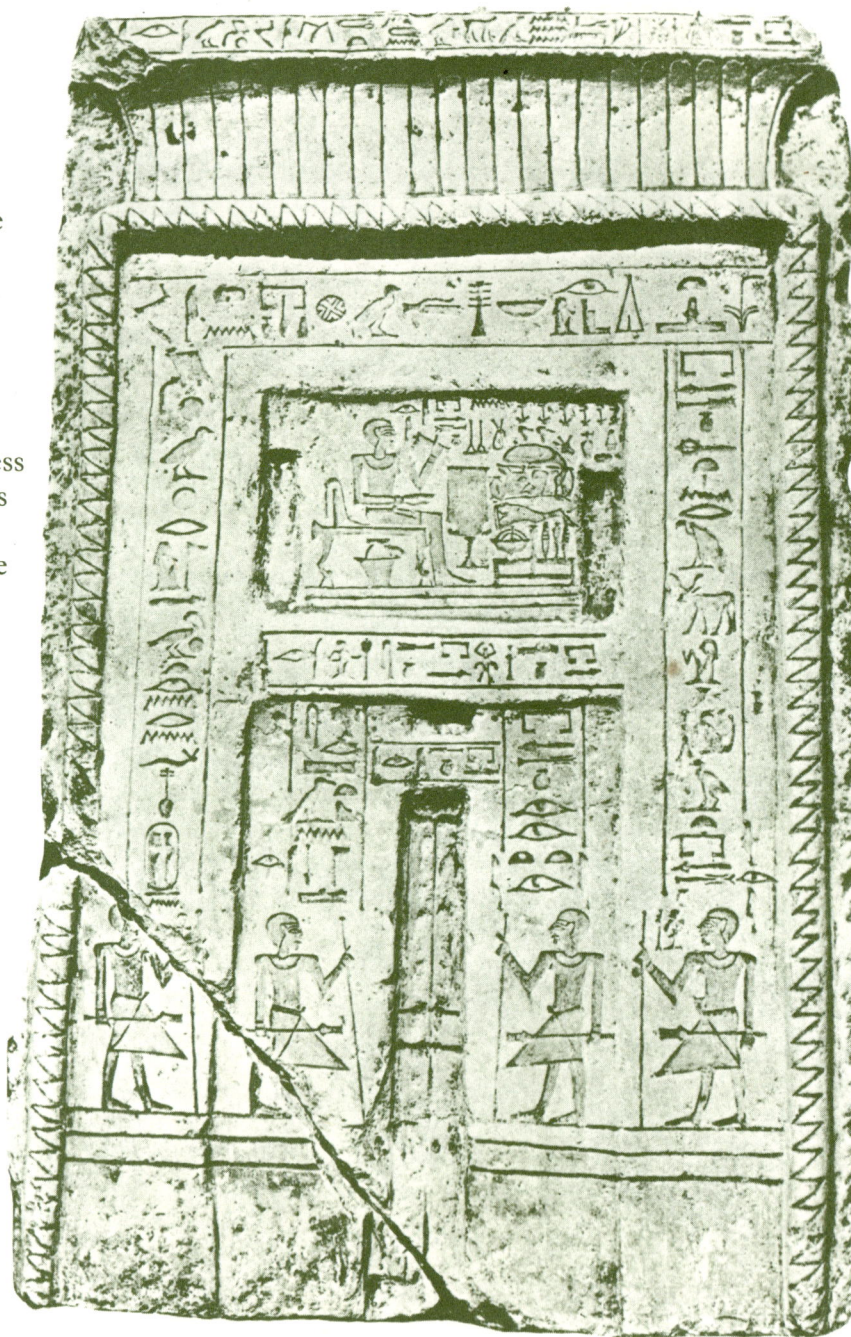

Funeral inscription to Irj, a physician at the Pharaoh's court. Irj lived about 1500 B.C. This inscription describes him as:
'Palace doctor
Superintendant of the court physicians
Palace eye physician
Palace physician of the belly
One understanding internal fluids
Guardian of the anus'

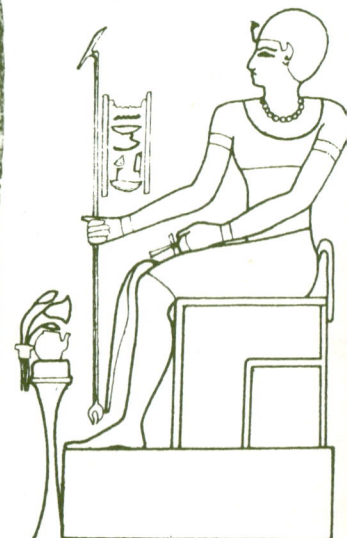

Imphotep, the vizier and physician of King Zozer, lived about 2600 B.C. and was later worshipped as a god of healing

Spells and magical potions

We know something about the medical knowledge and skills of these physicians and priests because of the discovery of a number of Egyptian medical documents. These 'books' were written on papyrus between about 1900 and 1500 B.C. They contain both supernatural and common sense explanations for illness.

Where there was no obvious reason for an illness, many Egyptian doctors and priests believed the disease to be caused by spiritual beings. In such cases, doctors and priests often recommended spells and magical potions to drive out these spirits. Here are some of the remedies they used:

Spell to be said when drinking a remedy

Here is the great remedy. Come! You who drives out evil things from my stomach and my limbs. He who drinks this shall be cured just as the gods above were cured. This spell is really excellent—successful many times!

(Papyrus Ebers)

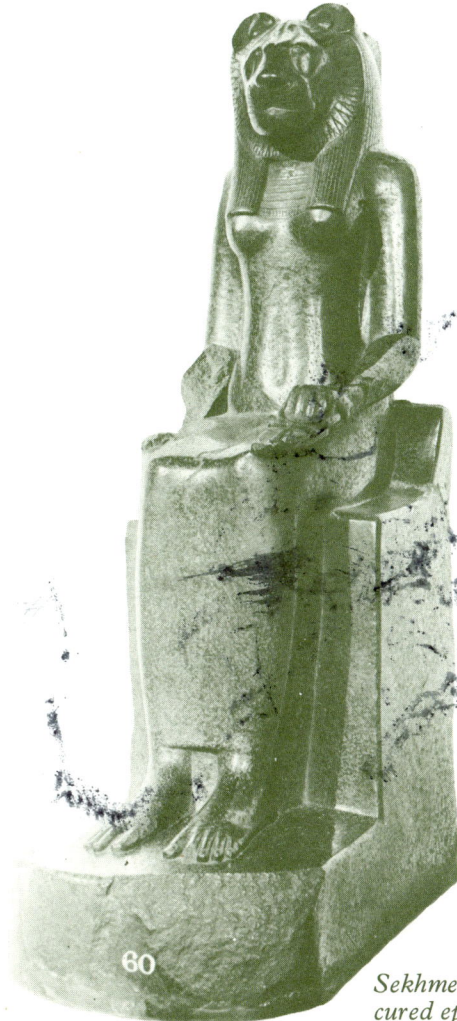

Remedies for a mother and child

These words are to be spoken over the sick person. 'O Spirit, male or female, who lurks hidden in my flesh and in my limbs, get out of my flesh! Get out of my limbs!'

(Papyrus Berlin)

Remedy to make the hair of a bald person grow

Fat of lion, fat of hippopotamus, fat of cat, fat of crocodile, fat of ibex, fat of serpent, are mixed together and the head of the bald person is anointed with them.

(Papyrus Ebers)

Sekhmet, the war goddess, who caused and cured epidemics

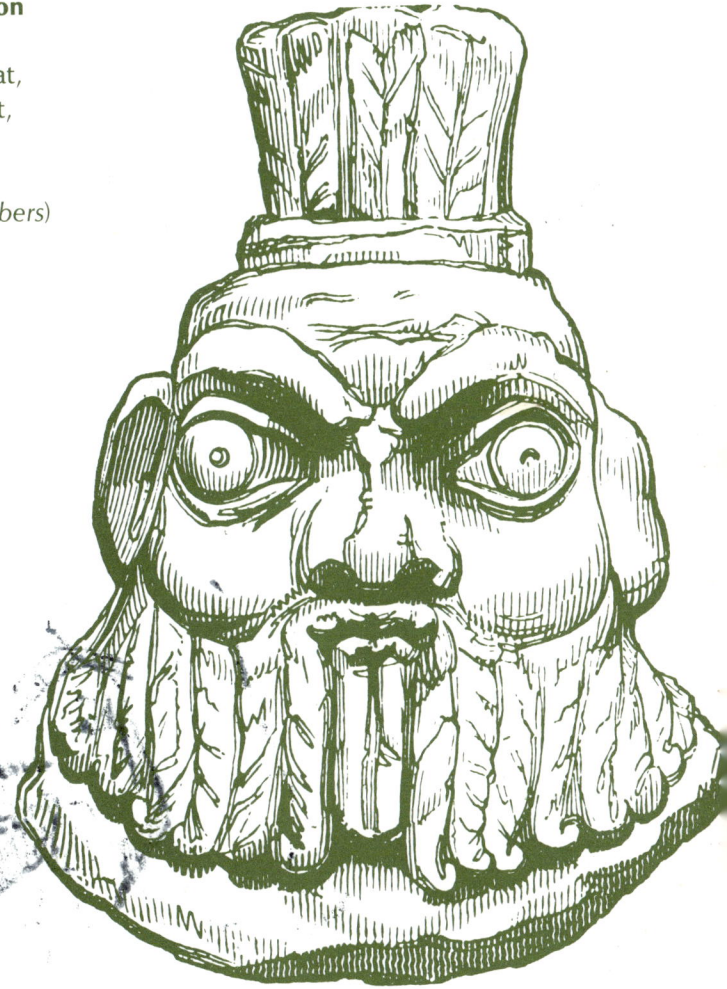

Bes, the god who frightened away evil spirits (redrawn from an Egyptian stone carving)

15

New knowledge about physiology

At the same time, many doctors and priests were beginning to develop different ideas about disease and its treatment. From the evidence of medical papyri, we know that Egyptian doctors had discovered certain things about the workings of the human body. As the extract below suggests, Egyptian doctors seem to have been aware that the heart, blood, air and even the pulse were important in some way to the workings of the human body. When Egyptian doctors wrote, 'His heart beats feebly', they knew it was an alarming symptom.

The Physician's secret: knowledge of the Heart, and the Heart's movements
(written about 1500–1600 B.C.)
46 vessels [channels] go from the heart to every limb. If a doctor, priest of Sekhmet or magician, places his hand or fingers on the back of the head, hands, stomach, arms or feet then he hears the heart. The heart speaks out of every limb.

There are: 4 vessels in his nostrils, 2 give mucus and 2 give blood.

There are 4 vessels in his forehead which then give blood to the eyes; all diseases of the eyes arise through them, because there is an opening to the eyes.

There are 4 vessels to the head . . .

There are 4 vessels to his 2 ears.   The breath of life enters into the right ear, and the breath of death enters into the left ear . . .

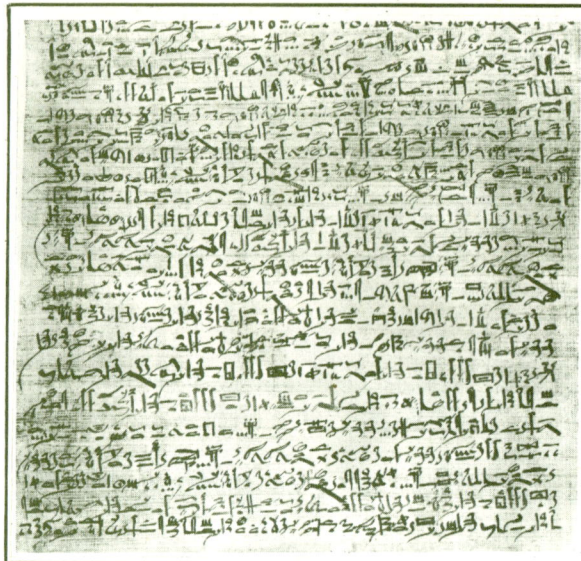

Column from a medical papyrus discovered in 1862 at Luxor by Edwin Smith, an American scholar

There are 6 vessels that lead to the arms . . .

There are 6 vessels that lead to the feet . . .

There are 2 vessels to his testicles; it is they which give semen.

There are 2 vessels to the buttocks . . .

There are 4 vessels to the liver; it is they which give to it humour and air, which afterwards cause all diseases to arise in it by overfilling with blood.

There are 4 vessels to the lung and to the spleen; it is they which give humour and air to it.

There are 2 vessels to the bladder; it is they which give urine.

There are 4 vessels that open to the anus; it is they which cause humour and air to be produced for it. Now the anus opens to every vessel to the right side and to the left side in arms and legs when [it] is overfilled with excrements.

(*Papyrus Ebers*)

New knowledge about anatomy

As the above extract shows, Egyptian doctors both knew about and had names for the main internal organs of the body such as the heart, liver, spleen and lungs. They seem to have believed that these organs were all connected to each other either directly or through the heart. Moreover, from a description of the brain in the *Edwin Smith Papyrus*, it is obvious that this organ had also been closely observed.

Perhaps doctors became aware of some of these organs when they treated open wounds. They may also have learned some details from the embalmers who preserved dead bodies.

Herodotus, a Greek traveller visiting Egypt in the 5th century B.C., described the process of embalming:
First they take a crooked piece of metal and with it draw out some of the brain through the nostrils and then rinse out the rest with drugs. Next they make a cut along the side of the body with a sharp stone and take out the whole contents of the abdomen.

After this they fill the cavity with myrrh, cassia and other spices and the body is placed in natron for 70 days.

(*Herodotus* Book 2 chapter 86)

The heart was usually left inside the body but the other internal organs were removed, treated with preserving spice, and placed in a canopic jar which was taken to the tomb

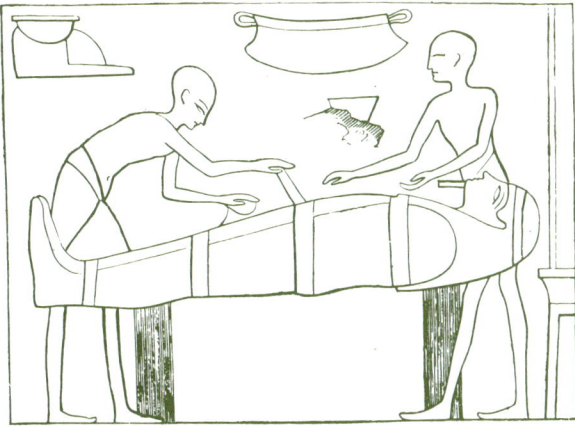

Egyptian embalmers bandaging a mummy (from a wall painting)

Remedy for blindness

A pig's eye, stibium, red ochre and a little honey are finely ground and mixed together and poured into the ear of the man so that he may be cured at once. Then recite this spell twice: 'I have brought this ointment and applied it to the trouble spot and it will remove the horrible suffering. Do this and you will see again.' A really excellent remedy!

(Papyrus Ebers)

with the mummy. Because of the heat, the process had to be carried out speedily. The embalmers were prevented not only by time but also by religious laws from examining the body in great detail.

The Egyptians believed that after death, the soul left the body for a time but that it returned shortly afterwards. From this moment a second existence would begin which was very similar to the first life. In this after-life, a man would need all his earthly possessions including his body. This is why the Egyptians felt that they must mummify their dead to preserve the body from decay. It also explains why they were forbidden to dissect and examine the limbs and organs, for this would prevent a man from enjoying the after-life.

As a result, Egyptian doctors seem to have had little knowledge of certain anatomical details, as the following remedy for blindness suggests:

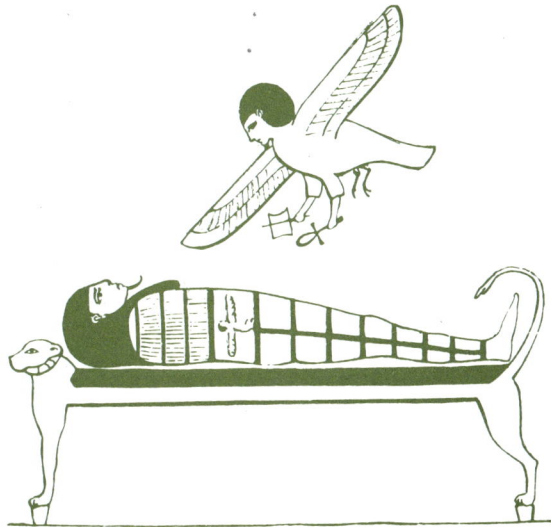

Tomb painting showing a soul returning to a body

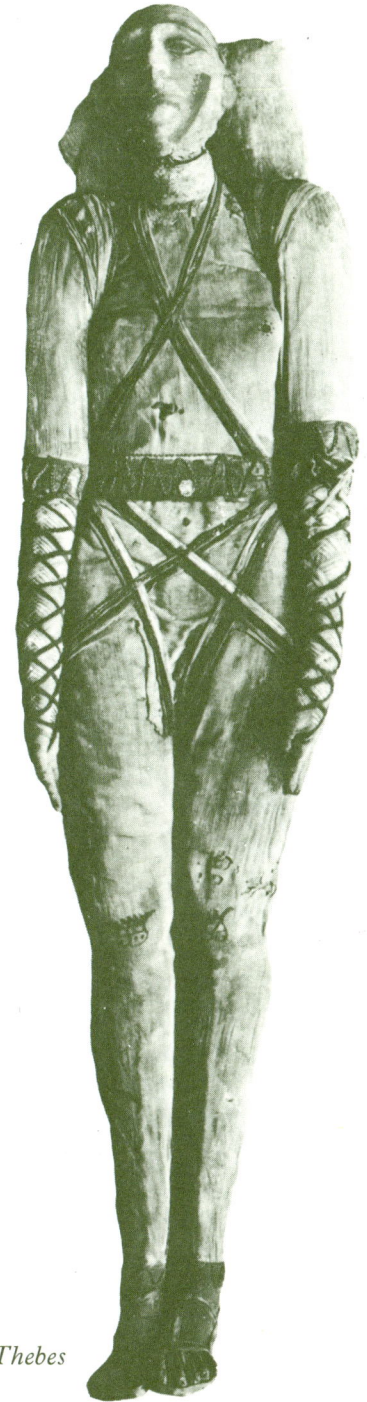

Mummy of an unnamed person found at Thebes

17

Examination and diagnosis

The observations of Egyptian doctors did not end with anatomy and physiology. According to the evidence of medical papyri, they also examined their patients carefully before diagnosing and treating their ailments.

Funeral inscription carved about 2000 B.C.

I was a priest of Sekhmet strong and skilful in the Art;
One who put his hands upon the sick and so find out;
One who is skilful with his eye.

Instructions for treating a broken nose

EXAMINATION

If you examine a man whose nose is disfigured—part of it being squashed in, while the other part is swollen and both his nostrils are bleeding.

DIAGNOSIS

Then you should say 'You have a broken nose and this is an ailment which I can treat.'

TREATMENT

You should clean his nose with 2 plugs of linen and then insert 2 plugs soaked in grease into his nostrils. You should make him rest until the swelling has gone down, you should bandage his nose with stiff rolls of linen and treat him with lint every day until he recovers.

(Papyrus Edwin Smith)

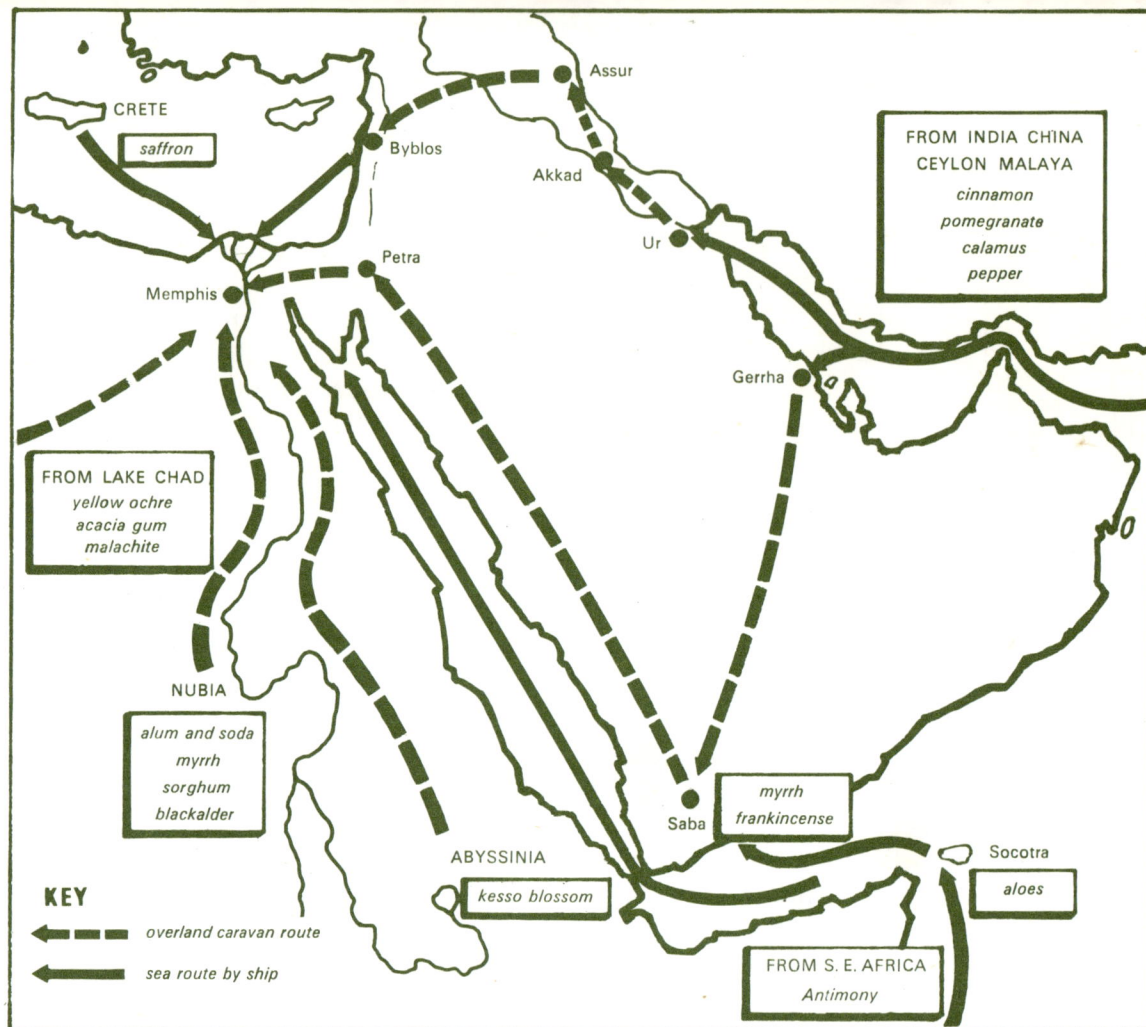

Map showing the Egyptian spice trade

CRETE
saffron

Byblos

Assur

Akkad

Ur

FROM INDIA CHINA CEYLON MALAYA
cinnamon
pomegranate
calamus
pepper

Petra

Memphis

Gerrha

FROM LAKE CHAD
yellow ochre
acacia gum
malachite

NUBIA

alum and soda
myrrh
sorghum
blackalder

Saba

myrrh
frankincense

Socotra
aloes

ABYSSINIA
kesso blossom

FROM S. E. AFRICA
Antimony

KEY

- - → overland caravan route

—→ sea route by ship

Treatment using herbs and drugs

Egyptian doctors developed a wide range of practical remedies and treatments which had no connection with spells or magical potions. Remedies based on herbs, plants, minerals, and animal parts were widely and successfully used to treat certain illnesses. Such drugs must have been considered to be of the greatest importance because minerals and plants were brought to Egypt from all over the known world.

Over the centuries the physicians must have observed which drugs were most effective against certain diseases and, aided by the invention of writing, they built up a store of knowledge which was based on experience.

So accurate was this knowledge that one third of these Egyptian medicinal plants were still used until recent years. Indeed modern chemists have even discovered germ-destroying substances in

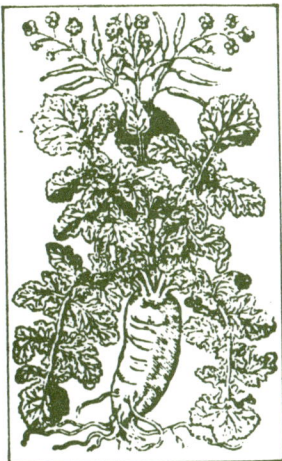

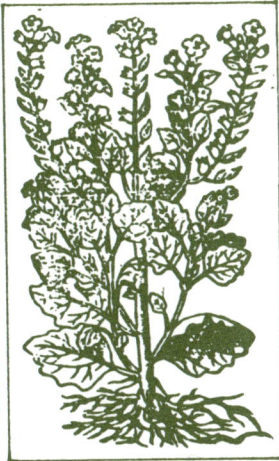

A radish : vast quantities of these together with garlic and onions were given to the workmen building the pyramids as payment in kind. Modern chemists have discovered that they all contain chemicals effective against dysentery, typhoid and cholera

Egyptian henbane used to 'still pain caused by worms in the intestines'. Modern chemists have discovered that it contains scopolamine which numbs certain nerves

some of the popular ingredients of Egyptian medicine such as myrrh, yeast (which was used in beer), mud, animal liver and animal dung.

Here are some remedies listed in the *Ebers Medical Papyrus*. Notice how the ingredients in one of these prescriptions were carefully weighed beforehand:

A remedy when the belly is ill
Cumin ½ ro, goosefat 4 ro, are boiled, strained and taken.
Another remedy, figs 4 ro, sebesten 4 ro, sweet beer 20 ro.

For a diseased eye
To clear up the pus: honey, balm from Mecca and gum ammoniac.
To treat its discharge: frankincense, myrrh, yellow ochre.
To treat the growth: red ochre, malachite, honey.
For diseases of the bladder
Bread in a rotten condition. The doctor must use it to fight the sickness—not to avoid the sickness.
For night blindness
Liver of ox, roasted and crushed out.
Really excellent!

(*Papyrus Ebers*)

Surgery

Herbs and drugs were not the only remedies prescribed by Egyptian physicians. By the same process of observation and trial and error they had acquired skills in using simple but effective treatments for wounds and dislocations.

One medical papyrus contains a description of an infected wound and recommends willow leaves as a treatment:

When you examine a man with an irregular wound and that wound is inflamed . . . and that man is hot in consequence; then you must say; 'A man with . . . a sickness I can treat.' Then you must make cooling substances for him to draw the heat out [with] leaves of willow.

Today, it is well known that solutions made from the leaves and bark of the willow contain antiseptic substances.

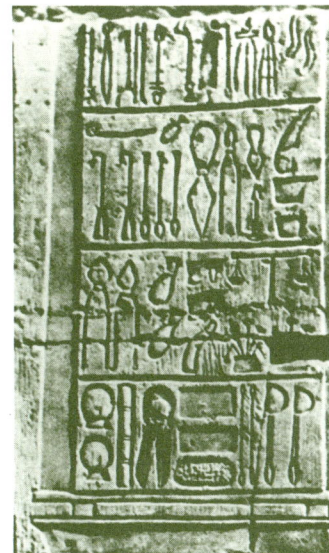

This stone carving from the temple of Kom Ombo is thought, by some historians, to show Egyptian surgical instruments

Although there is no evidence of major internal operations, we do know that simple surgery was carried out on cysts and tumours. Notice how the physician carefully examined his patient beforehand and noted other symptoms:

Instructions for examining swellings in the body
When you come across a swelling of the flesh in any part of the body of a patient and your patient is clammy and the swelling comes and goes under your finger except when your finger is still, then you must say to your patient, 'It is a tumour of the flesh. I will treat the disease. I will try to heal it with fire since cautery heals.'

When you come across a swelling that has attacked a vessel, then it has formed a tumour in his body. If when you examine it with your fingers, it is like a hard stone, then you should say, 'It is a tumour of the vessels. I shall treat the disease with a knife.'

(*Papyrus Ebers*)

A 'new' theory about the cause of disease

Besides the use of herbs, drugs and surgery we also have evidence that doctors recommended treatments involving purging, vomiting and bloodletting.

These treatments seem to have been connected with a 'new' theory about the cause of certain diseases. This theory shows that Egyptian doctors did not believe that all diseases were caused by spirits.

Just as the Nile and its irrigation channels watered the land of Egypt, so Egyptian doctors seem to have viewed the human body as a system of channels (or vessels). If the irrigation canals were out of order then the land suffered. Similarly, certain diseases would result if the internal channels of the body became blocked by blood or mucus or food. When such blockages were thought to have happened then doctors prescribed remedies to clear them:

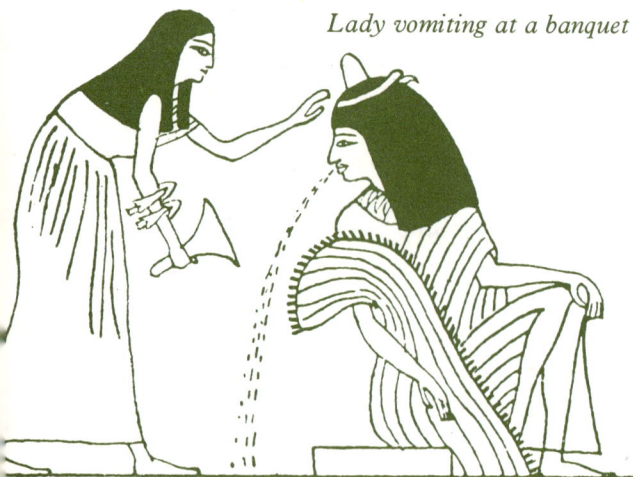

Lady vomiting at a banquet

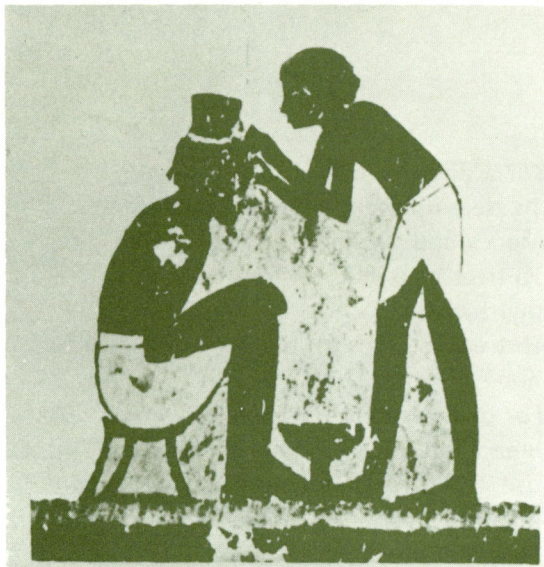

This tomb painting may show a surgeon (or barber) applying blood sucking leeches to a patient

The collection on the expelling of the wehedu

There are 2 vessels in him to his arms; if he is ill in his arm . . . then thou shalt say concerning it: one suffering from . . . let him vomit by means of fish and beer and his fingers are bandaged with water melon until he is healed.

(*Papyrus Ebers*)

To clear the bowels after a blockage

Colocynth, senna, fruit of sycamore are ground, mixed together and shaped into 4 cakes and let him eat it.

(*Papyrus Ebers*)

Instructions for treating inflammations

Remedy for curing the disease: Let him be rubbed with pumice stone till the swelling subsides.

Another remedy: let him be given the knife treatment on the lower thigh.

(*Papyrus Ebers*)

From evidence recorded by Herodotus in the fifth century B.C., it seems likely that the Egyptians also used purges to preserve health as well as to cure sickness:

For three following days in every month they purge themselves . . . for they think it is from the food they eat that all sicknesses come to men.

(*Herodotus* Book 2, chapter 77)

This idea about the cause of disease was of course an unproved theory. Nevertheless it shows that Egyptian doctors had begun to look for natural rather than supernatural explanations for the cause of disease.

Ideas about health

The Egyptians were not only interested in medicine and disease, they were also interested in health. Many people believed that the best way to remain healthy was to scare away the evil spirits which brought disease, so they wore charms. Scarab beetles were thought to be particularly effective and elaborate jewelled brooches and pendants were made in this shape for the rich.

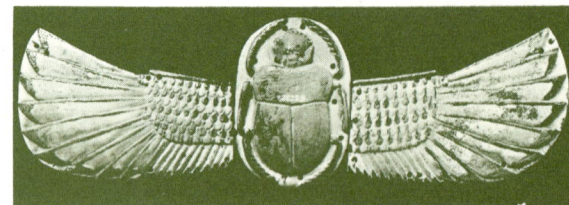

Jewelled charm in the shape of a scarab beetle

More homely charms were used by the poor, such as this one recorded in a medical papyrus, made by a mother to protect her child:

I have made a charm for my child which will protect him against you, oh evil spirits! This charm is made from evil smelling herbs and from garlic which is harmful to you; from honey which is sweet for men and horrible for spirits, from a fish tail and a rag and a backbone of a perch.

(*Papyrus Berlin*)

At the same time, however, the Egyptians seem to have devised more rational methods of preserving health and preventing disease.

Herodotus made the following observations:

Gnats are abundant, this is how the Egyptians protect themselves against them . . .

Each man possesses a net. By day it serves him to catch fish, while at night he spreads it over the bed . . . and . . . goes to sleep underneath. The gnats, which if he rolls himself up in . . . a piece of muslin, are such to bite through the covering, do not so much as attempt to pass the net.

(*Herodotus*, Book 2, chapter 93)

Egyptian hygiene

The Egyptians were also very concerned about their personal hygiene and this too helped to protect their health. Herodotus was very impressed by the Egyptians' elaborate 'code' of hygiene when he visited Egypt in the fifth century B.C.

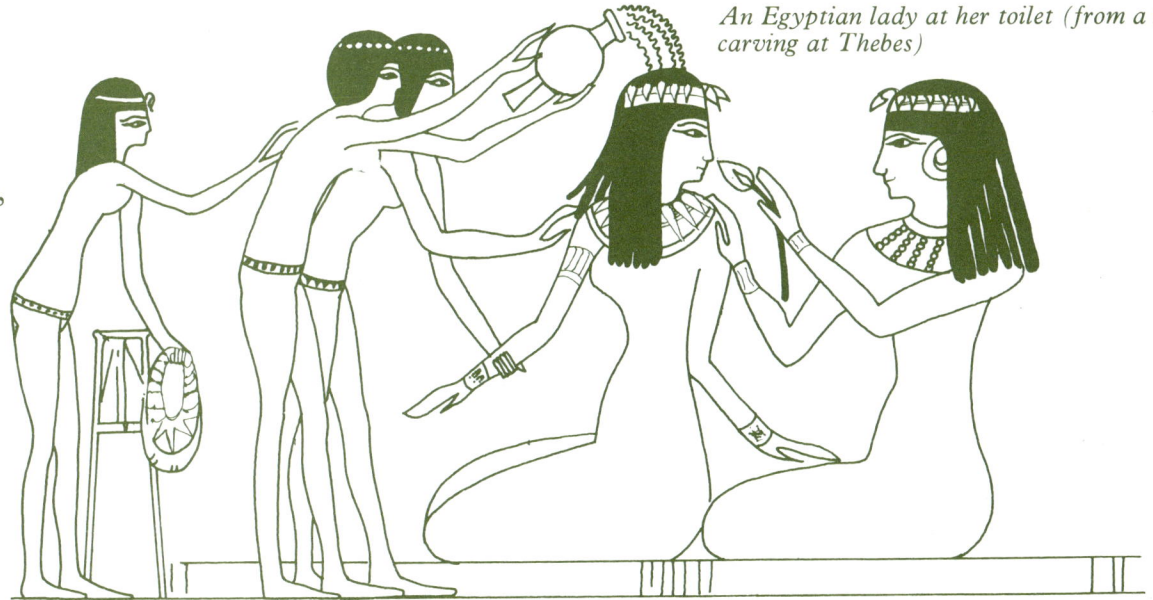

An Egyptian lady at her toilet (from a tomb carving at Thebes)

They are especially religious—more than any other nation; and these are some of their customs.

They drink from cups of bronze which they clean daily and this is done not just by some people but by everyone. They are especially careful always to wear newly washed linen clothing. They practise circumcision for the sake of cleanliness . . . . Their priests shave the whole body every third day so that no lice . . . may infest them while they are in the service of the gods . . . Twice a day and every night they wash in cold water.

Pigs are thought by the Egyptians to be unclean animals. If an Egyptian touches a pig in passing by, he goes to the river and dips himself in it fully clothed. Moreover, of all Egyptians, only swineherds are forbidden to enter any temple. No Egyptian will give his daughter to a swineherd in marriage . . . and so swineherds intermarry amongst themselves.

(*Herodotus* Book 2, chapters 37 and 47)

Not only the priests but also ordinary people, both rich and poor, washed frequently in the morning and evening and before every meal. Soda, scented oil and ointments were used as soap. Ointments were considered so important that they formed part of the payments in kind made to workers in place of wages.

It is interesting to note that Herodotus connects the Egyptians' 'code' of hygiene with their religious practices. Some modern historians have suggested that the religious and hygienic laws of the Jews were influenced by the Egyptian 'code'. Moses and the Israelites had no doubt learned of Egyptian practices during their years of captivity in Egypt.

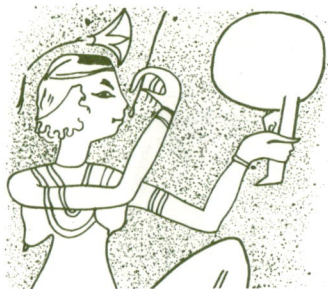

An Egyptian lady painting her lips (from a drawing on papyrus)

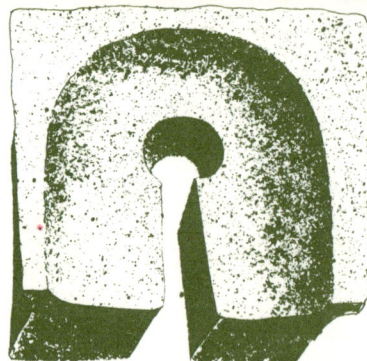

Limestone latrine seat

Egyptian ladies were not only concerned about their personal hygiene, they also took great care over their appearance. They shaved their bodies with bronze razors, and anointed their skin with oils and perfumes. Lips, cheeks and eyes were skilfully painted. Lead sulphide and 'soot from the wall' were mixed with goose fat to make black eye make-up. Powdered emerald-green copper ore was also used to make green eye shadow. These cosmetics, however, were probably applied not only for the sake of vanity, but because the Egyptians had also discovered from experience that they helped to protect the eyes from the many infectious eye diseases common at this time.

Although many rich people had bathrooms in their homes, the plumbing was very simple. There were no tubs, only limestone slabs with a low rim around them, where the bathers sat and had water poured over them from a jug. The waste water was carried off by a little gully which disappeared through a hole in the wall and drained into a sunken vase in the floor which was emptied afterwards.

Simple toilets or latrines have also been discovered in Egyptian houses. These consisted of a limestone seat with a vase in a pit beneath. Though the Egyptians had learned much about using water to irrigate the fields they had not begun to use it for flushing and cleansing of drains.

Some conclusions

From the study of medical papyri and other evidence we can tell that by 1500 B.C. the Egyptians had already acquired a great deal of sound knowledge about medicine and hygiene.

By the fourteenth century B.C. Egyptian doctors were so famed for their skill that they were loaned to foreign courts in Syria and Assyria. We know this from a number of diplomatic 'letters' between Egyptian and neighbouring rulers which were recorded on clay tablets and stored in the royal archives at Tel-el-Amarna.

In the seventh century B.C., the Greek writer Homer commented that, "In medical knowledge the Egyptians leave the rest of the world behind."

A little later Egyptian doctors may even have met and exchanged ideas with Greek physicians. The Greeks are sometimes thought to have been the first doctors to use 'scientific' approaches to medicine, yet it is clear that 1000 years before the Greeks, Egyptian doctors had already become skilled at observing and examining their patients, and had also developed rational explanations for the cause of disease. Indeed, it seems likely that the Greeks learned a great deal about medicine from the Egyptians.

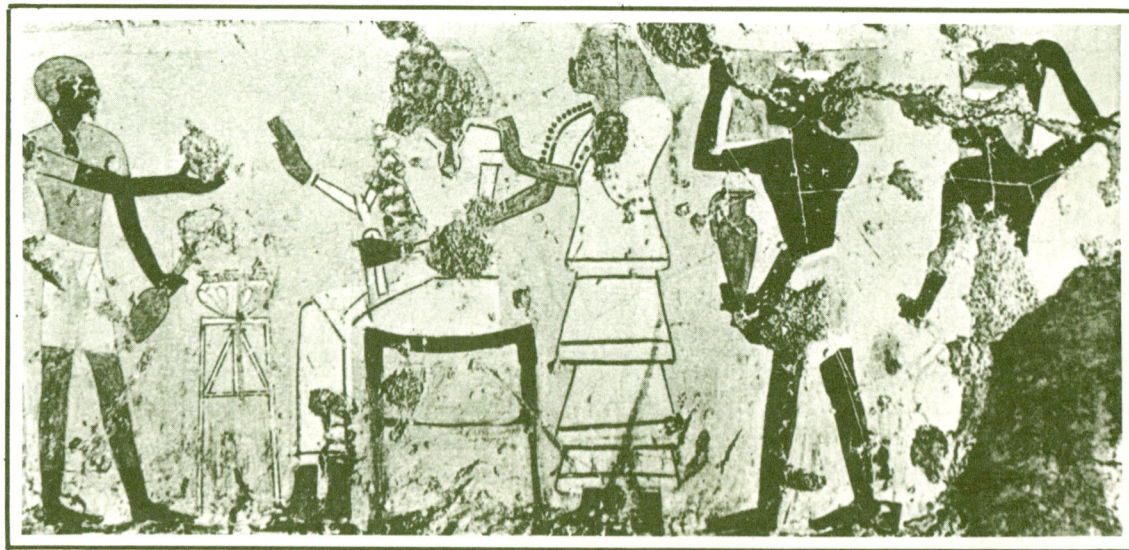

Wall painting showing a Syrian prince (seated) consulting the Egyptian physician Nebamon. The physician is holding a bottle and handing a potion to his patient

3. The Greeks and medicine

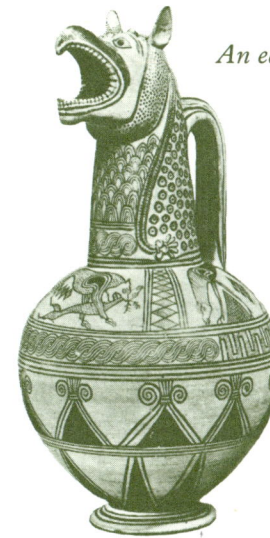

An early Greek jug (700–650 B.C.)

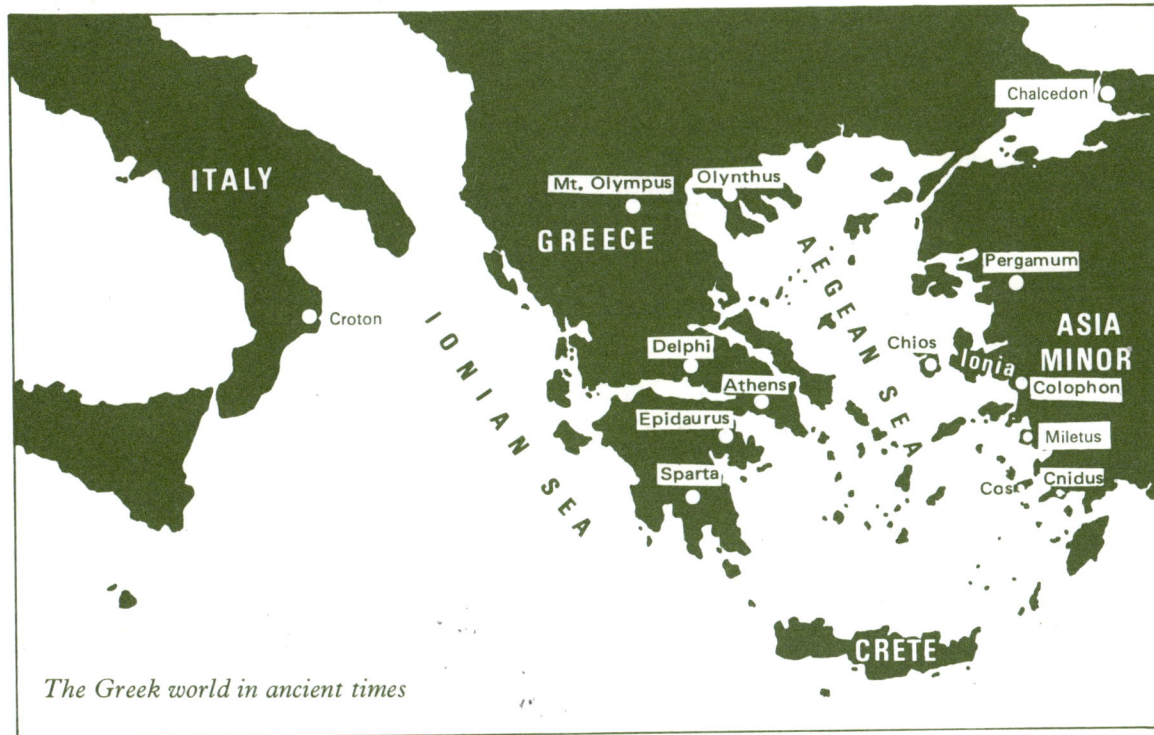

The Greek world in ancient times

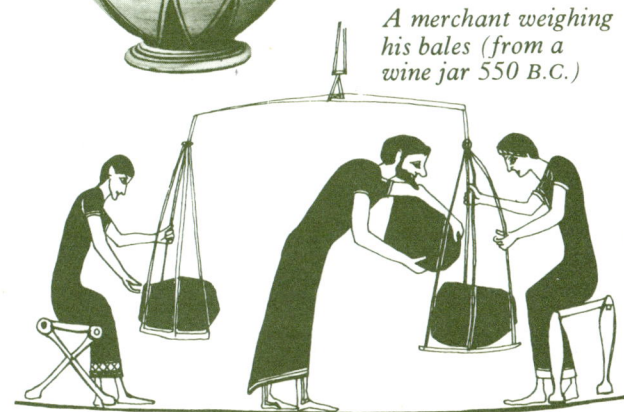

A merchant weighing his bales (from a wine jar 550 B.C.)

The early Greeks, 1600–700 B.C.

From 1600 B.C. onwards, when the Egypt of the Pharaohs was flourishing, the Greeks too were beginning to develop their own civilisation. Our information about their beginnings is scanty but we do know that they lived together in small, walled villages. From 1600–1200 B.C. they seem to have been ruled by kings and chiefs who lived in palaces and were buried surrounded by rich possessions in beehive shaped tombs cut into the hillside. After 1200 B.C. the towns and villages were governed for the next 100–700 years by councils of the most important men.

Farming had developed, and like the Egyptians, the Greeks no longer spent all their time gathering food and seeking shelter. Craftsmen were making jewellery and weapons from bronze, and pottery decorated with beautiful and complicated designs. There were sailors, traders and merchants who kept records in a primitive kind of writing. According to legend, in 776 B.C. the first Olympic Games were held. The Greeks had time to spare for war as well as sport and music. Metal workers made elaborate armour for their soldiers.

In time, the early Greeks increased their knowledge about the world and developed many skills and crafts. Like the Egyptians, however, they also worked out supernatural explanations for many of the common facts of nature.

According to the mythology of the early Greeks, the sea was governed by a god named Poseidon who lived in a golden palace beneath the Aegean sea. It was Poseidon who whipped up the waves causing white horses to leap up from the foam. He lifted

23

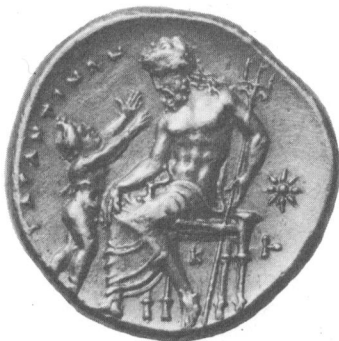
Greek gold coin, 340–330 B.C. showing the god Poseidon

Machaon bandaging the leg of Menelaus
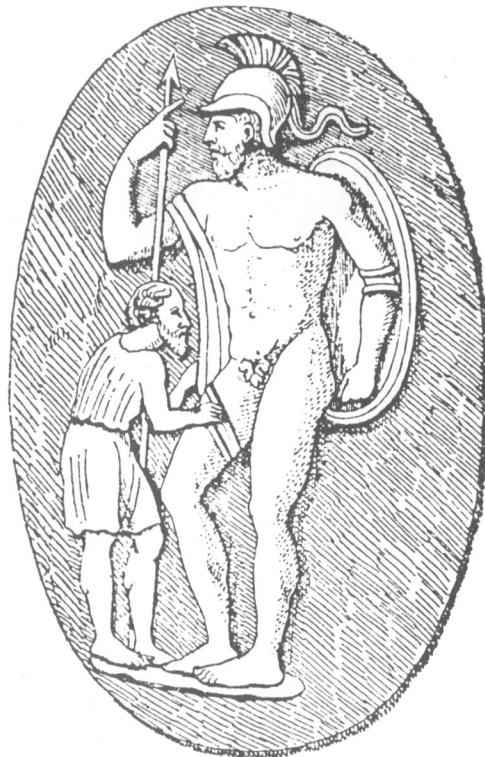

up ships, causing wrecks, and when he struck the ground with his trident the earth would quake or springs would burst from the rocks.

Volcanoes, on the other hand, were the workshops of Hephaestos, the god of fire. Here, according to legend, Hephaestos forged iron and worked as a blacksmith. People could see the smoke from his furnace and the sparks from his anvil coming out of the

top of the volcano. In its rumblings they could hear the roar of his bellows and the sound of his hammer.

Winter, spring and summer were brought by the goddess Demeter. Her daughter Persephone had been carried off by the god of the underworld and was allowed to spend only six months of each year with her mother. While Persephone was away, Demeter was sad and in her anger she would allow no crops to grow or flowers to bloom and winter covered the land. When her daughter returned, however, Demeter was content once more and spring came. The trees began to blossom and the crops to grow again.

Early Greek medicine

As with the Egyptians, the medicine of the early Greeks reflected their beliefs about the world in general. We know from the writings of the poet Homer that the Greeks were practising medicine around 1000 B.C. In his poem about the Trojan wars, the *Iliad*, Homer described many of the wounds received by the Greek warriors. We learn how the Greek leader Menelaus was injured by an arrow and how Machaon the doctor-in-arms tried to pull it out. When the arrow-head broke off, Machaon sucked the blood from the wound and applied a soothing ointment. This was in fact a simple but effective treatment for a wound based on experience and common sense.

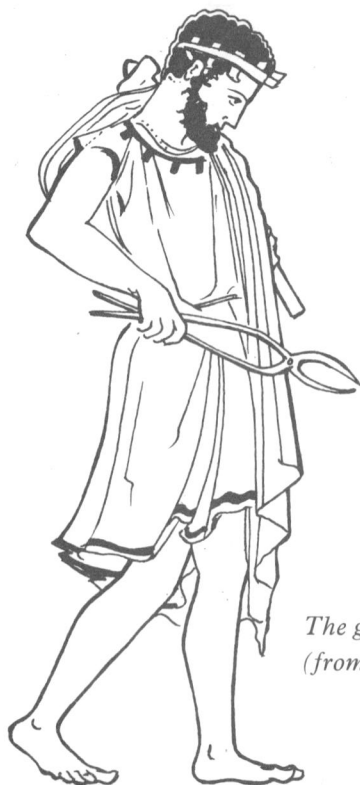
The god Hephaestos (from a Greek vase)

By the eighth century B.C., we have evidence of a different aspect of Greek medicine. It seems that by this time many sick people were making the journey to consult the oracle of the god Apollo at Delphi about their ailments.

Asclepios and temple medicine

By the sixth century B.C., many Greeks seem to have turned to Asclepios, a legendary hero-turned-god, to heal and cure them. Temple-sanatoria called *Asclepeia* were built in quiet places. Here people came to bathe, sleep, meditate and beg Asclepios to cure them. As you will see from the extract below, serpents played an important part in this cult.

Aristophanes, a Greek who lived between about 450–385 B.C., wrote a play in which he described how Plutus, the god of wealth, visited an *Asclepeion* in the hope of regaining his sight. His servant describes the visit:

Statue of Asclepios

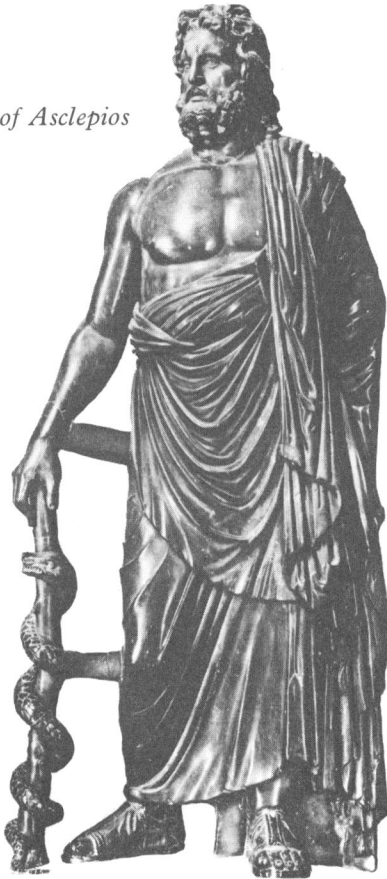

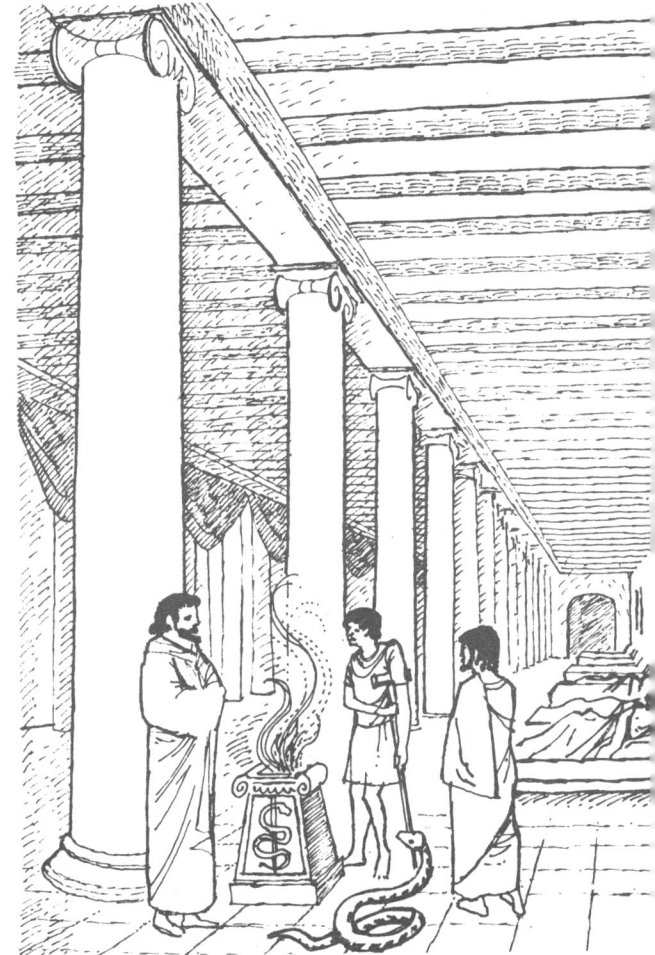

First we had to bathe Plutus in the sea. Then we entered the temple where we placed our offerings to the gods on the altar—honey cakes and sweetmeats. There were many sick people present, with all kinds of illnesses. Soon the temple priest put out the light and told us all to go to sleep and not to speak no matter what noises we heard . . .

(from *Plutus: the god of riches*)

The place where the patients slept was called the *abaton*, a long building with a roof supported by columns and with open sides. The Greeks believed that while the patients were asleep they were visited by Asclepios and his daughters, Panacea and Hygeia. Plutus' servant described how his master was cured by them:

The god went round with calm and quiet steps to every patient looking at each disease. Then by his side a servant placed a stone pestle and mortar and a medicine chest. First he mixed an ointment for Neoclides, a blind man, by crushing together garlic, verjuice and squills and adding vinegar. This ointment he placed on the man's eyes. Then he sat down by Plutus. First he wiped the patient's head, then with a cloth of clean linen he wiped Plutus' eyelids a number of times. Next Panacea covered his face and head with a scarlet drape. The god whistled and two huge serpents appeared. They crept under the scarlet cloth and licked his eyelids. Then

Plutus sat up and he could see again but the god, his helpers and the serpents had vanished.

(from *Plutus*)

In the morning the sick were supposed to wake up cured. We know that many people were cured because they left inscribed stones

Restoration of the interior of the abaton at the Asclepeion at Epidaurus

25

as thanksgiving offerings to the gods. Here are the words carved on two of these votive stones:

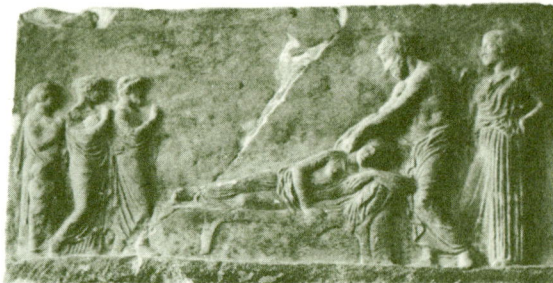

> Hermodicus of Lampsacus was paralysed in body. When he slept in the temple the god healed him and ordered him to bring to the temple as large a stone as he could. The man brought the stone which now lies before the abaton.

> Agestratos was unable to sleep on account of headaches. As soon as he came to the abaton he fell asleep and had a dream. He thought that the god cured him of his headache and, making him stand up, taught him wrestling. The next day he departed cured, and after a short time he competed at the Nemean games and was victor in the wrestling.

Some people were not miraculously cured overnight and for them the temples became more of a health resort and place of convalescence, as the plan of part of the *Asclepeion* at Epidaurus shows. These *Asclepeia* remained important centres of rest and healing for many hundreds of years. People continued to visit them even when other ideas about medicine developed. The Romans were impressed by the cult of Asclepios and during the third century B.C. these ideas spread to Italy.

Restoration of the area around the Asclepeion at Epidaurus

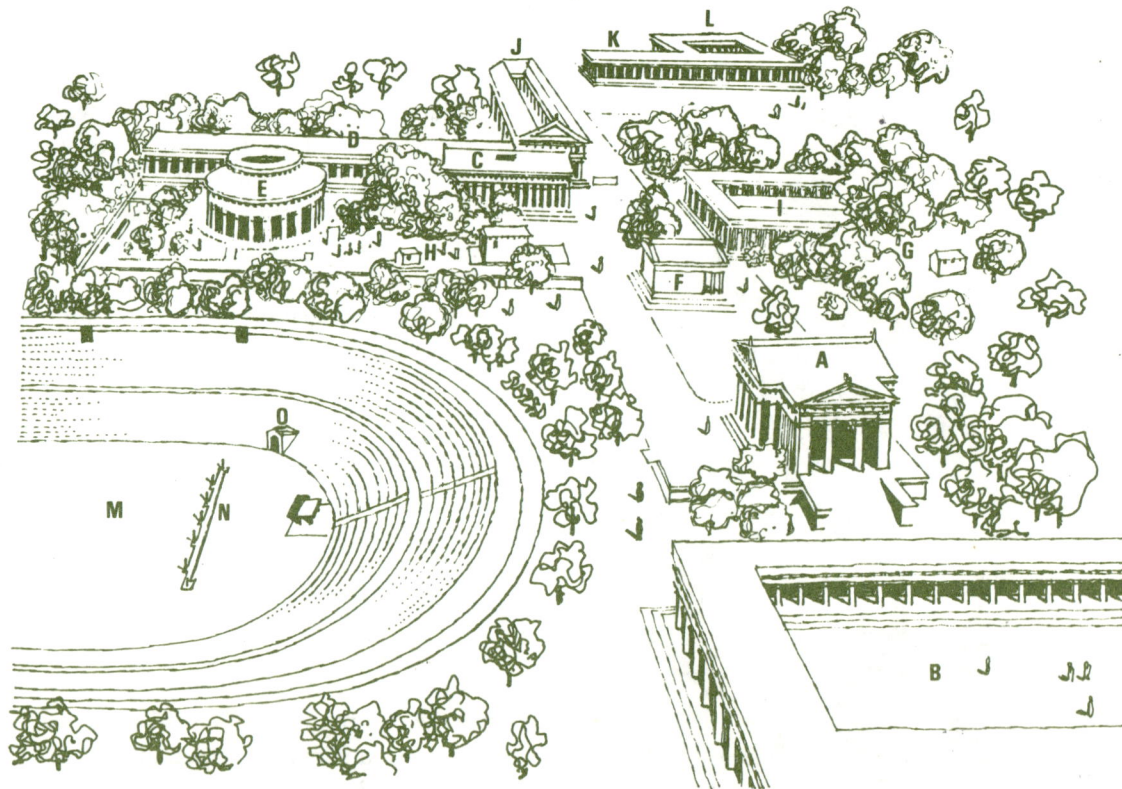

KEY *to the most important buildings*
A *South propylaea* B *Gymnasium* C *Temple of Asclepios* D *East and west abaton* E *Tholos* F *Temple of Artemis* G *Grove* H *Small altar* I *Square building* J *Baths of Asclepios* K *North eastern colonnade* L *North eastern quadrangle* M *Stadium* N *Goal* O *Tunnel*

The Greeks and Greek philosophy 600–400 B.C.

In the sixth century B.C. other developments were taking place which were also to affect Greek medicine. At this time certain Greek thinkers began to develop more rational explanations for many of the happenings in the world of nature. Their theories were to have an important influence on ideas about health and medicine.

Most of these Greek thinkers (or *philosophers* as they were called) came from the Ionian islands or Greek cities and colonies on the coast of Asia Minor and southern Italy. We cannot say precisely why people from these places first began to develop a new kind of interest in the world. Perhaps they were influenced by the place and time in which they lived. Their cities were on trades routes used by merchants and travellers from the Near and Far East, and many Greeks in these cities came into contact with the ideas and beliefs of the Egyptians and people from other lands. The Greeks may have learnt a great deal from Egyptian ideas about mathematics, geometry and medicine, but it is unlikely that they simply copied the ideas of the Egyptians. As sailors and island people, many of the Ionian Greeks had long been close observers of the natural world. Knowledge of the wind, the weather and the stars was very important for navigation. As traders, many Greeks had learned much about the geography of the Mediterranean lands.

Knowledge gained from the Egyptians perhaps combined with their own

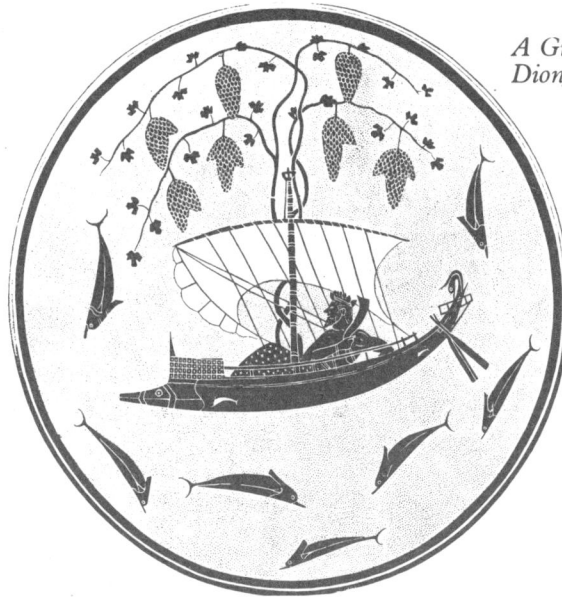

A Greek ship sailed by a larger than life Dionysus, god of wine (from a bowl, 500 B.C.)

observations and became food for further thought. As a result the Greeks developed an approach to science which differed slightly from that of the Egyptians, as some historians have pointed out:

> The Greeks . . . [were] . . . not content with recording the practical arts [e.g. building, irrigation etc.] . . . [They] began to look at the world as a whole and tried to see a pattern in it, to discover reasons why it was such as they thought it to be. Thus, about 600 B.C., began *theoretical* science intended to fulfil the desire to *know*, rather than the desire to achieve.
> (from *An illustrated history of science* by F. Sherwood Taylor, Heinemann 1955, pp. 1–2.)

Whatever the reasons, during the sixth century B.C. Greek philosophers began to develop new theories about the origins of the world and natural life. These theories were arrived at by a process of logical reasoning and observation and without the aid of myths and legends.

Thales of Miletus (c. 585 B.C.) was one of the earliest Greek philosophers. He was also a practical scientist who busied himself with the solution of many technical problems. Thales was concerned with the first of many important questions about the world which were to interest other Greek philosophers— *What are things made of?* According to tradition Thales had visited Egypt and seen how the flood waters fertilised the land. His interest in these floods, however, went beyond that of many Egyptian scholars. They applied their knowledge of mathematics and geometry to the practical problems of constructing irrigation channels and controlling the flood waters.

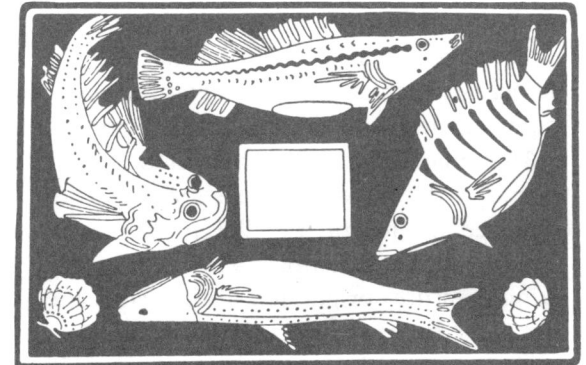

Four fish and two shells are shown on this plate of baked clay produced by a Greek artist in southern Italy in the 4th century B.C. Aristotle, the Greek philosopher who also lived at this time, made a detailed study of sea creatures

Thales, however, became interested in the question of the importance of water to all human, plant and animal life. He came to the conclusion that water was one of the basic elements in all things.

Anaximander, another Greek philosopher (c.560 B.C.), also came from Miletus. He was interested not only in water but also in fire, earth and air, which he believed to be the other basic elements in all things. Anaximander concluded that thunder and lightning were not the work of the god Zeus, but were caused in a perfectly natural way when air, which had been compressed in a cloud, burst out with great force.

The idea that all things in the world were made of four basic elements was accepted and developed by many other Greek philosophers. Each of the four elements was thought to have a different quality. Fire was hot and dry, air was hot and moist, water was cold and moist, earth was cold and dry. Theories about these four qualities and the elements which shared them were to have an important influence on Greek medicine.

Anaximander was also interested in the second of the important questions asked by the Greek philosophers—*Where do things come from?* Anaximander believed that all living creatures originated in the water and that some became land animals when the water evaporated. Human beings too, originally came from fish-like creatures.

Pythagoras (c.530 B.C.) was a Greek philosopher who lived for many years in Croton in southern Italy. He investigated the world of nature and came to the conclusion that all things had some mathematical relationship to each other. Pythagoras became particularly interested in the idea of balance and opposites, not only in mathematics but in matters of health. Pythagoras and his followers believed that health was a state of perfect bodily balance. They tried to lead a life of moderation in all things so that this balance would not be upset.

Many of the ideas of these philosophers mark the beginning of sciences such as physics and biology. This does not mean that Greek philosophers no longer believed in the existence and importance of gods. When Thales was asked if there was a place for gods in his theories about the world, he is reported to have replied, "all things are full of gods". Greek philosophers were merely trying to show that some things had natural rather than supernatural explanations. The ideas and methods of these philosophers had important effects when they were applied to medicine.

Hippocrates and the new ideas about medicine

By about 460 B.C. it seems that Greek doctors from the Ionian islands and the coast of Asia Minor were beginning to investigate problems of health and disease by a process of reasoning and observation.

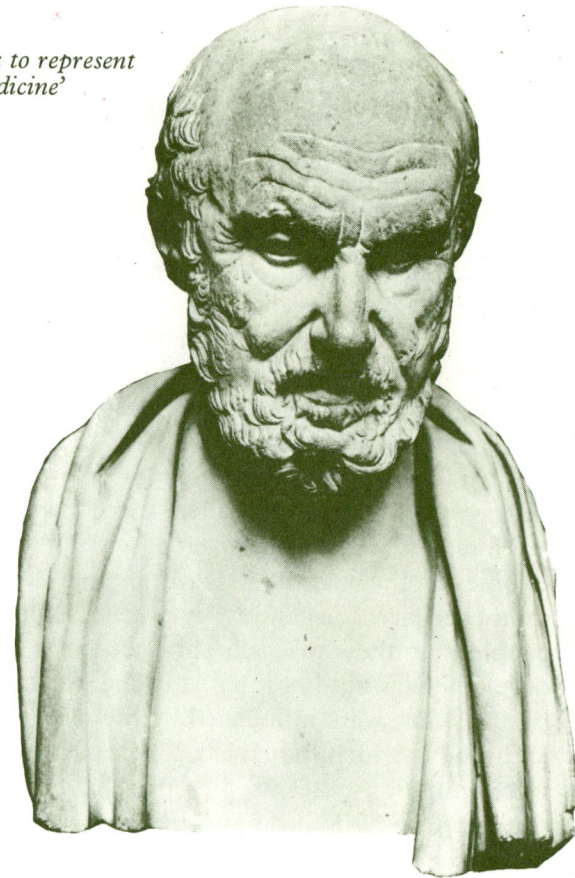

Hippocrates of Cos

The most famous of these Greek physicians was Hippocrates. Actually we know very little about him as a person. The earliest biographies were written a long time after his death and so they are probably not very reliable. However, he is mentioned by Plato and Aristotle who lived at the same period, so we can assume that he did exist.

His biographers claim that Hippocrates was born on Cos, an island near the coast of Asia Minor, about 460 B.C. We do know something about the work of Hippocrates and other Greek doctors at this time, through a collection of over sixty medical 'books'. Scholars have shown that only a few of these were written by Hippocrates himself. The remaining books were written over the next 150 years by other Greek doctors, many of whom had similar ideas. These books became known as the Hippocratic collection.

Hippocrates and the clinical method of observation

Hippocrates and other Greek doctors believed that the art of the physician should be separated from the cult of the priest. The physicians, they believed, should try and discover natural explanations for disease by studying their patients. Egyptian doctors had examined their patients but Hippocrates and other doctors insisted that all patients should be more systematically observed and the results recorded. Indeed, this method of 'clinical observation' is, with modifications, still used today. These ideas were to turn doctors from miracle healers into clinical scientists and they have earned Hippocrates the title, 'The Father of Medicine'.

Some of the books in the Hippocratic collection give detailed advice about how doctors should examine their patients:

First of all the doctor should look at the patient's face. If he looks his usual self this is a good sign. If not, however, the following are bad signs—sharp nose, hollow eyes, cold ears, dry skin on the forehead, strange face colour such as green, black, red or lead coloured. If the face is like this at the beginning of the illness, the doctor must ask the patient if he has lost sleep, or had diarrhoea, or not eaten.
(from *On forecasting diseases* section 2)

During an illness all the patient's symptoms were noted:

Silenus had become overtired from drinking and exercising at the wrong time and had caught a fever. He began with pains in his abdomen, heavy head and a stiff neck.
First day: he vomited, his urine was black, he was thirsty, tongue dry, no sleep at night.
Second day: slightly delirious.
Third day: symptoms worse.
Sixth day: slight perspiration about the head; head and feet cold and livid, no discharge from the bowels, no urine, acute fever.
Eighth day: cold sweat all over, red rashes, severe diarrhoea, urine bitter and passed with pain, hands and feet cold.
Eleventh day: he died—breathing slow and heavy, stomach throbbing. His age was about twenty.
(from *On epidemics* Book 1, case 2)

By carefully examining their patients and recording their symptoms, Hippocrates and other doctors found that they could set out a natural history of the illness. This could then be used to forecast the development of the illness in future cases. This, they believed, was very important:

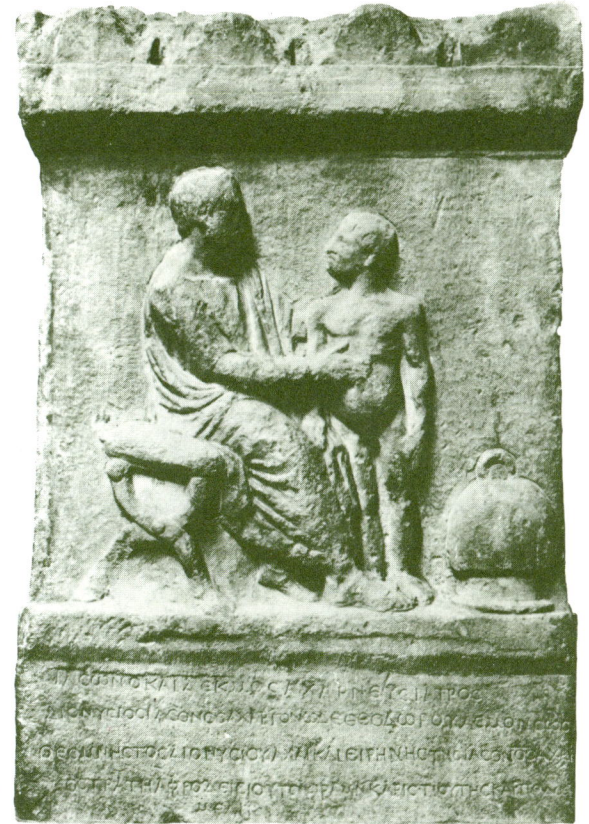

I believe that it is an excellent thing for a physician to practise forecasting. He will carry out the treatment best if he knows beforehand from the present symptoms what will take place later.
(from *On forecasting diseases*, section 1)

These ideas about the importance of accurate and relevant observation of disease spread far and wide. Even Thucydides, the Greek historian, felt it was important to produce a detailed record of the symptoms and effects of the Great Plague which came to Athens in the summer of 430 B.C. Here are extracts from his description of the plague:

I shall describe what the plague was like, and set down the symptoms. I had the disease myself and saw others suffering from it. People in perfect health suddenly began to have burning feelings in the head; their eyes became inflamed; inside their 'mouths there was bleeding, and the breath became unpleasant. The next symptoms were sneezing and hoarseness of voice, and before long the pain in the chest was accompanied by coughing. Next the stomach was affected with stomach aches and with vomiting of every kind of bile. Externally the body was not very hot to the touch: the skin was reddish and livid, breaking out into small pustules and ulcers. But inside there was a feeling of burning, so that people could not bear even the lightest linen clothing.

At the beginning the doctors were quite incapable of treating the disease because of their ignorance of the right methods . . .

Equally useless were prayers made in the temples, consultation of oracles, and so forth.

(*History of the Peloponnesian War* Book 2, chapters 47–54)

The natural causes of disease

Throughout their minute observations of their patients Greek doctors always worked on the assumption that disease had *natural* and not supernatural causes. Here is the view of one Greek doctor on the cause of epilepsy, thought to be a 'divine' or 'sacred' disease connected with the gods:

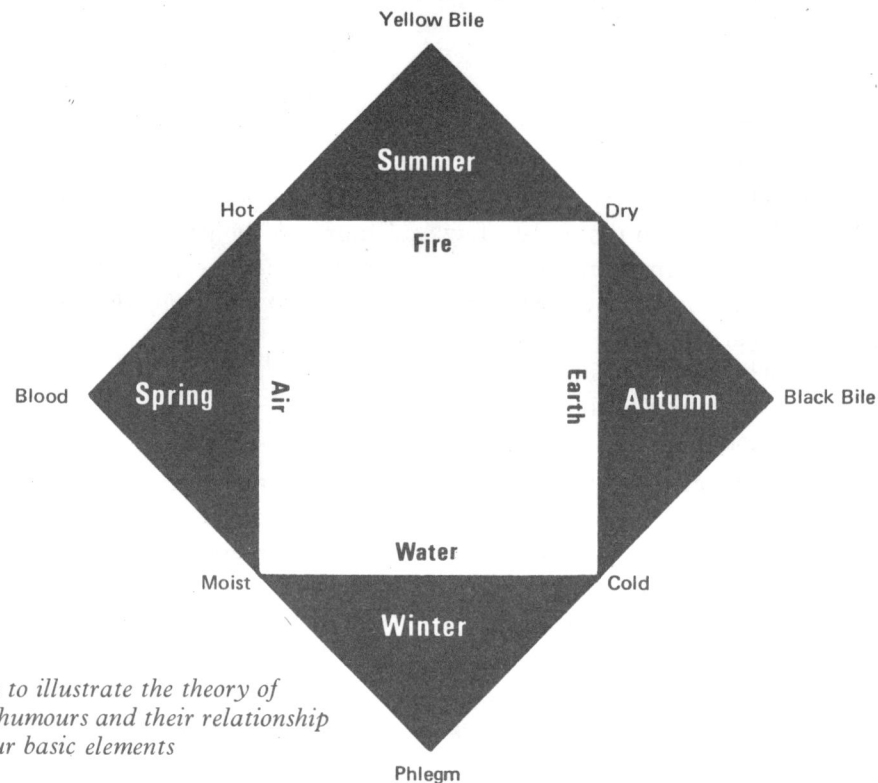

Diagram to illustrate the theory of the four humours and their relationship to the four basic elements

It is not, in my opinion, any more divine or sacred than other diseases are; there are natural signs (preceding the onset of the disease). Men believe only that it is a divine disease because of their ignorance and amazement . . .

(from a book on *The Sacred Disease*, section 1)

Unfortunately Hippocrates and other Greek doctors made little progress in investigating the cause of disease any further. They had, of course, no technical aids such as the microscope, but they do not seem to have shown a strong interest in the actual physical cause of disease. Many doctors did, however, accept a theory of the cause of disease which was based on the ideas of the philosophers about the four basic elements and the balance of health.

The theory of the four humours

This theory suggested that the body was made up of four liquids or 'humours', blood, phlegm, yellow bile and black bile. Doctors observed that when a man was sick one of these liquids was usually present. The patient might, for instance, be bleeding, coughing phlegm or vomiting bile. Doctors did not realise that the presence of these humours might be the *result* of an illness. They thought that the humours must, in some way, be the *cause* of the disease. Some doctors, therefore, came to the following conclusions:

Man's body . . . has blood, phlegm, yellow bile and melancholy bile [black bile]. These make up his parts and through them he feels illness or enjoys health. When all these elements [humours] are truly balanced and mingled, he feels the most perfect health. Illness occurs when one of these humours is in excess, or is lessened in amount or is entirely thrown out of the body . . . When one of these elements [humours] is isolated so that it has no balance . . . the particular part of the body where it is supposed to make balance, naturally becomes diseased.
(from a book *On the constitution of man*, section 4)

One question remained—what caused one liquid to increase more than another? Each humour, like the four elements, had its own quality and so was either cold, dry, hot or moist. The weather and the seasons were thought to have a definite influence on the humours. Phlegm, the coldest of the humours, increased in winter. At that time, therefore, phlegm diseases are more common and people can be seen sneezing and blowing their noses.

In spring, as the cold relaxes and the rains come on, blood increases for it is hot and moist like the spring. In spring dysentery and bleeding from the nose are common when people are hot and red. In summer blood is still strong but yellow bile increases

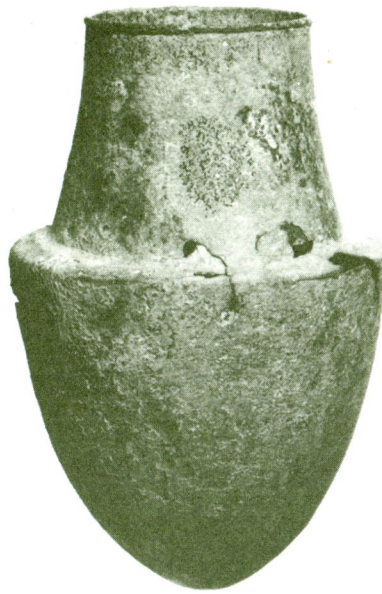

A bronze bleeding cup (115 mm high); these were heated and placed over a scratch made on the patient's back; as the cup cooled a small amount of blood was drawn off into it

until the autumn. During this time people vomit bile, become feverish and the skin is often yellow. Autumn is a dry season beginning to be cold and the black bile dominates in the body. Finally as winter approaches, black bile is chilled and reduced and gives way to phlegm.

Natural cures

Since diseases had natural causes, it seemed obvious to doctors that cures should also be natural. Greek doctors were convinced that "nature itself is the best healer" and that whenever possible, they should not interfere with this process. There were, however, some treatments which could help nature and the body's own "innate heat" to restore the humours to their correct balance.

Certain foods were thought to influence the humours:

I think that barley soup is better than all other cereal foods for chest diseases—also vinegar and honey for they bring up phlegm and quench thirst.
(from a book *On the treatment for acute diseases* section 10)

On other occasions doctors felt it necessary to bleed their patients if excess blood was thought to be the cause of the disease:

When there is pain in the side a good thing is to apply a big soft sponge dipped in water and squeezed out. If the pain spreads as far as the collar bone, open the vein near the elbow and take away blood till it flows much redder.
(from a book *On the treatment for acute diseases* section 21)

Bleeding cups were often used since this was a less extreme method than opening the veins with a knife.

Knowledge about herbs and drugs had reached the Greeks from Egypt and these too were used to purge the body of excess liquids. Baths were also thought to be an effective remedy in some cases:

If the pain is under the diaphragm, clear the bowels with a medicine made from black hellebore, cumin and anise or other fragrant herbs. A bath will help pneumonia as it soothes the pain and brings up phlegm. But the bather must be quiet. He must do nothing himself but leave the pouring of water and rubbing to others.
(from a book *On the treatment for acute diseases* section 23)

A programme for health

Most doctors, however, shared the general view of the Greeks and preferred to preserve health rather than to treat disease. Athletics and sport had been part of the Greek way of life for hundreds of years. Stadia and gymnasia were built all over Greece. Sport formed part of the education of all Athenian boys between the ages of six and fourteen. Boys were placed in the charge of a trainer who kept a palaestra or exercise ground, which consisted of a central courtyard covered by sand, dressing rooms and baths. There the boys were instructed in running, jumping, discus and javelin throwing, wrestling and boxing. They exercised in the nude after anointing with oil as a protection against the sun. Afterwards they scraped the sand off with a special instrument, then bathed. Gymnasia and palaestra often seem to have had shower baths, similar to those in the picture on p. 33.

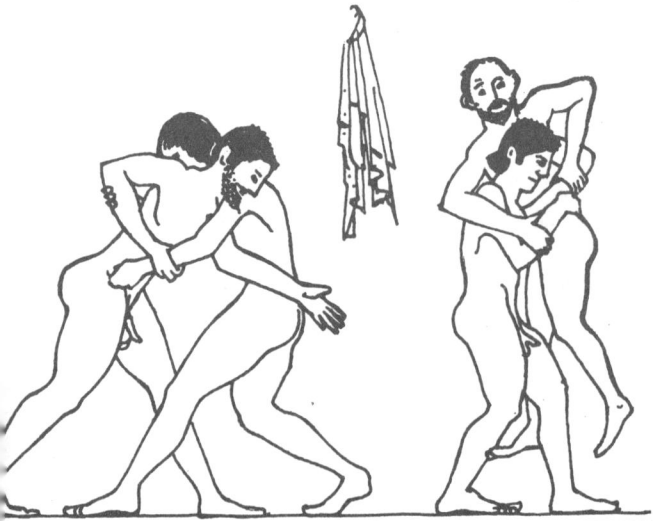

Running man (from a Greek amphora)

The Hippocratic collection contains *A programme for health*. The programme aimed at keeping the body at an even temperature and so ensuring that extremities of heat or cold did not unbalance the four liquids in the body. Correct food and exercise were the most important aspects of this programme:

> A wise man should consider that health is the greatest of human blessings. In winter, people should eat as much as possible and drink as little as possible— unwatered wine, bread, roast meat and few vegetables. This will keep the body hot and dry. In summer they should drink more and eat less—watered wine, barley cakes and boiled meat so that the body will stay cold and moist. Walking should be fast in winter and slow in summer.
>
> (from *A programme for health* sections 1, 8, 9)

We also possess a very interesting document which probably describes what Hippocrates and other Greek physicians considered a day spent in healthy living. It is a fragment from a book written by Diocles of Carystus, a famous physician who lived at Athens toward the end of the fourth century B.C. He lived later than Hippocrates but views on hygiene had hardly changed during the century. The fragment is too long to be quoted in full and the following extract is shortened and paraphrased in parts:

> The cultivation of health begins with the moment a man wakes up. A young or middle-aged man should take a walk of about 10 stadia just before sunrise. After awakening he should not arise at once but should wait until the heaviness of sleep has gone. After arising he should rub the whole body with some oil. Thereafter he should every day, wash face and eyes with the hands using pure water. He should rub his teeth inside and outside with the fingers using some fine peppermint powder and cleaning the teeth of remnants of food. He should anoint nose and ears inside, preferably with well-perfumed oil. He should rub and anoint his head every day but wash it and comb it only at intervals.
>
> After such a morning toilet, people who are obliged or choose to work will do so, but people of leisure will first take a walk. Long walks before meals clear out the body, prepare it for receiving food and give it more power for digesting.

Such elaborate personal hygiene required time and leisure. It was the hygienic way of life which could be led only by a rich citizen whose sole occupation was politics

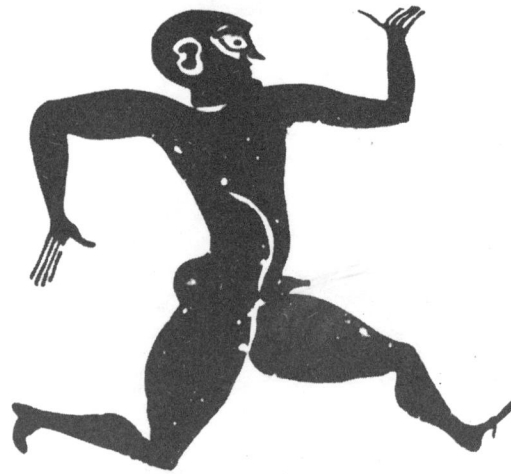

Wrestlers (from a Greek vase)

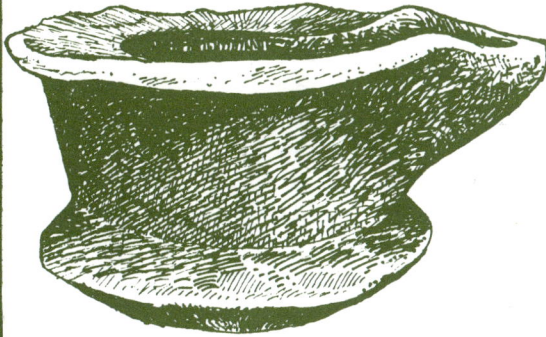
Terracotta toilet seat from Olynthus

In contrast to the magnificent public buildings such as the temples and gymnasia, the houses in the cities seem to have been poor places by comparison. A traveller from Asia Minor who visited Athens at the end of the 3rd century B.C. commented: "the city of Athens has a poor water supply and is badly divided into streets. Its houses are so cheap that a stranger entering the city for the first time would hardly believe it was the famous city of Athens". Archaeologists excavating the site of the ancient town of Olynthus in northern Greece have discovered terracotta bath tubs and latrines in houses of the wealthy. The poor seem to have used wash basins for bathing

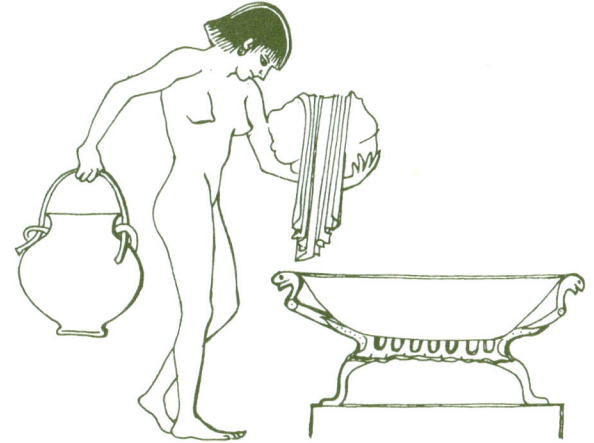
Girl preparing to wash (from a Greek cup 480 B.C.)

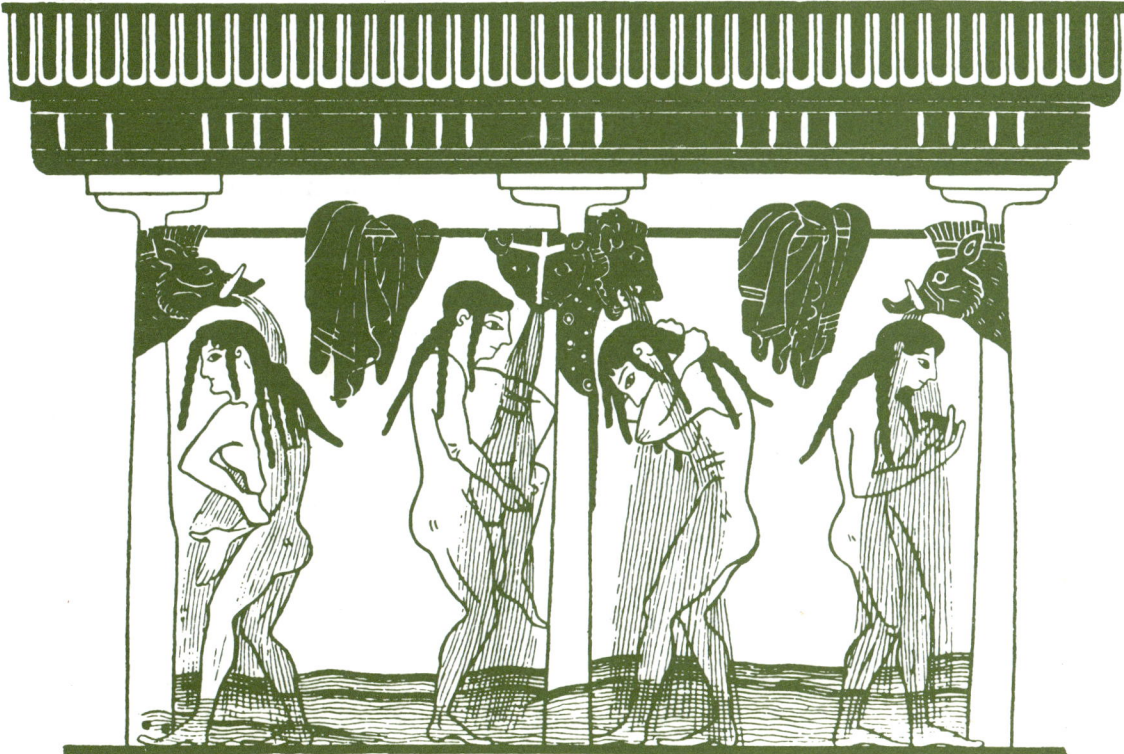
Greek women taking a shower bath (from a Greek vase sixth century B.C.)

and service to the state. The traders, craftsmen and farm labourers obviously could not afford to lead such a life. This was especially true of the slaves who had no control over their hours of work and rest or over their food.

The Hippocratic book *On Diet* has advice, "for the mass of people who drink and eat what they happen to get, and who are obliged to work to make a living, and who otherwise lead an irregular life". All they can do is consider the season in which they happen to be and try to adapt their meals and exercise to it as best they can. It is little enough but they are people who "by necessity must lead a haphazard life and who cannot take care of their health".

A code of behaviour

By Hippocrates' time Greek doctors were regarded as members of a skilled profession, and so a high standard of conduct was expected of them.

33

First they must be well trained:

He who is going to learn medicine and become a doctor must be intelligent and must be taught well from his childhood. (from a book of *Rules* section 2)

They were to be efficient and thoughtful:

A doctor must be able to remember all the drugs and their uses. You must prepare your medicine in good time. You must visit your patients often and must be careful when you examine them. When you enter a patient's room be calm and remember your bedside manners. Sometimes the patient may need scolding, sometimes comforting. (from a book *On Behaviour* sections 9–16)

They were to behave correctly towards their patients:

I will swear by Apollo, Asclepios and by all the gods that I will carry out this oath. I will use treatment to help the sick according to my ability and judgement but never with a view to injury or wrongdoing. I will not give poison to anybody . . .
. . . I will be pure and holy in my life and practice. Whatever I see or hear professionally or in my private life which ought not to be told I will keep secret.

This promise became known as *The Hippocratic Oath* and this oath is still taken today in a modified form at some medical schools.

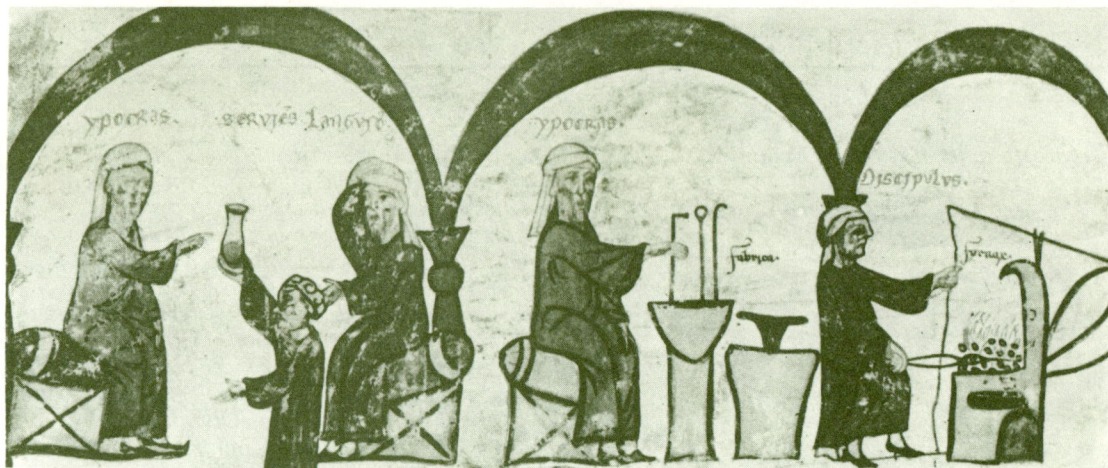

Hippocrates studying a patient's urine held up in a flask by a servant. The patient is sitting on the right (from a thirteenth-century copy of Hippocrates' works)

The making of surgical instruments

Surgery and anatomy

Despite the growth of these new ideas on the cause and treatment of disease, during Hippocrates' time Greek doctors recorded little new information in their books about the anatomy and physiology of the human body. It is possible that Greek doctors were, at this time, forbidden by religious beliefs to dissect dead bodies and examine the internal organs.

In the fourth century B.C., however, the philosopher Aristotle dissected many animals and gave good descriptions of certain internal organs such as the stomach and the womb. Although their knowledge of human internal organs was therefore limited, some Greek doctors made careful observation of the bone structure and the skull when treating injuries and fractures to the skeleton. Some doctors and surgeons became expert at treating displaced limbs, jaws, and fractured bones. They took great care to ensure that broken arms and legs did not mend in a deformed way and even attempted to straighten curved spines. Surgical operations on the inner parts of the body were not, however, attempted.

Greek medicine at Alexandria

It was not until after Hippocrates' time that Greek doctors began to study the anatomy of the body in detail. By 300 B.C. many Greeks, following the ideas of the philosophers Plato and Aristotle, came to believe that the body was not important after death and that only a person's spirit lived on. As a result Greek doctors at last were free for a time to dissect human bodies and study their structure and workings.

The most famous of these doctors worked at Alexandria in Egypt. In 335 B.C. Egypt had been conquered by a Greek army led by Alexander the Great and now Egypt was ruled by one of Alexander's generals— a man named Ptolemy. He made Alexandria his capital and wished to make it also the most famous city in the world. He built a great museum and library and invited the most famous writers, thinkers and doctors to come and work there.

In Alexandria the study of medicine became very important. Physicians began to go beyond the work of Hippocratic doctors and make new discoveries about the structure and workings of the body. Herophilus travelled from Chalcedon in Asia Minor and came to study in Alexandria. He became one of the first men to dissect bodies in public. He discovered that the brain (and not the heart, as Aristotle believed) controlled all movement in the body. Another Greek, Erasistratus, came to Alexandria from Chios. He came near to discovering the circulation of the blood. This new knowledge encouraged doctors to practise surgery and many complicated surgical instruments were gradually devised.

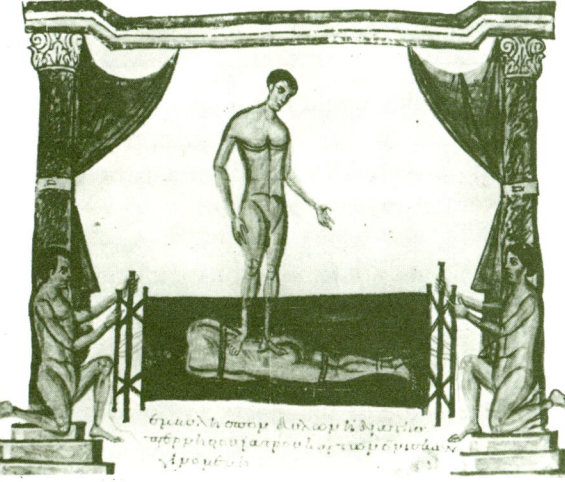

A method of treatment for displaced vertebrae in the spine (from a commentary by Apollonius of Kition on the works of Hippocrates)

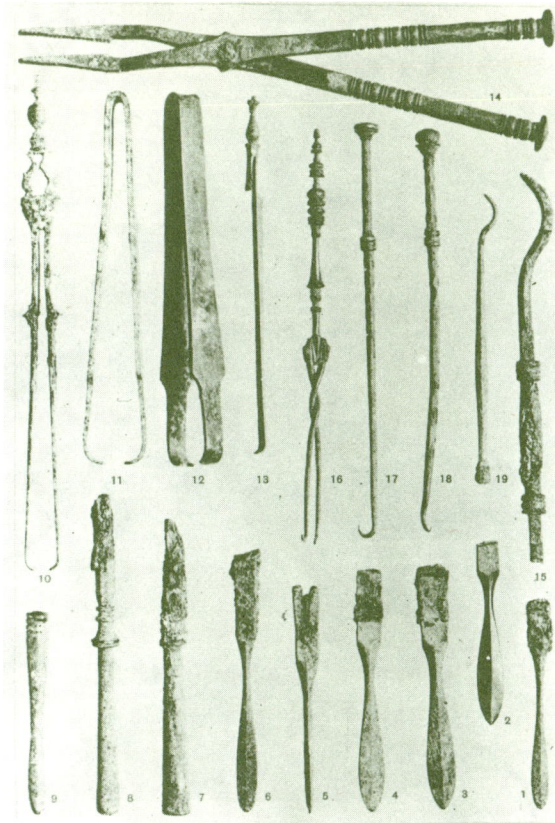

A set of Greek surgical instruments found at Colophon, Ionia (from Journal of Hellenic Studies, *vol. 34 : 1914)*

The Greeks and scientific medicine: some conclusions

After 460 B.C. Greek doctors such as Hippocrates developed many important ideas about medicine, disease and health. It has sometimes been said that Greek doctors 'set scientific medicine on its course', and in some ways this is true.

Certainly many Greek doctors, like modern doctors, believed that medicine should be based on knowledge of the patient and his or her symptoms gained through observation. At the same time, however, we must remember that the methods of Greek doctors were not exactly the same as those of modern scientists, as one historian has commented:

Though the Greeks created rational medicine [i.e. medicine based on reason and observation] their work was not always or even fully scientific in the modern sense of the term. In the investigation of living things, the complexity of . . . fact is so great that nothing can be established without constant observation . . . [and] . . . experiment, to determine what is normal and healthy and what is abnormal and diseased. Like other Greek pioneers of science, the physicians were prone to think that much more can be discovered by mere reflection and argument than is in fact the case.

(from *Greek Medicine* by E. D. Philips, Thames & Hudson 1975, p. 14)

Moreover, the Greeks were not the first to realise the importance of observing and examining patients, as we already know. Finally, we must not forget that the *Asclepeia* continued to play an important part in the treatment of many sick people both during and after the time of Hippocrates. The medicine of the healing temple and of Hippocrates developed side by side.

4. The Romans and the beginnings of public health

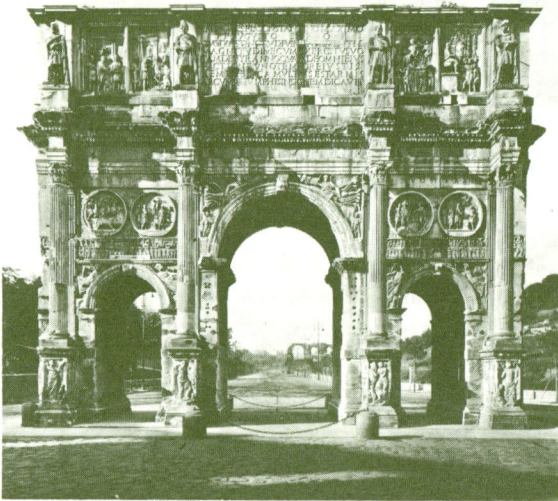

The triple arch of the Emperor Constantine, built in Rome (312–15 A.D.)

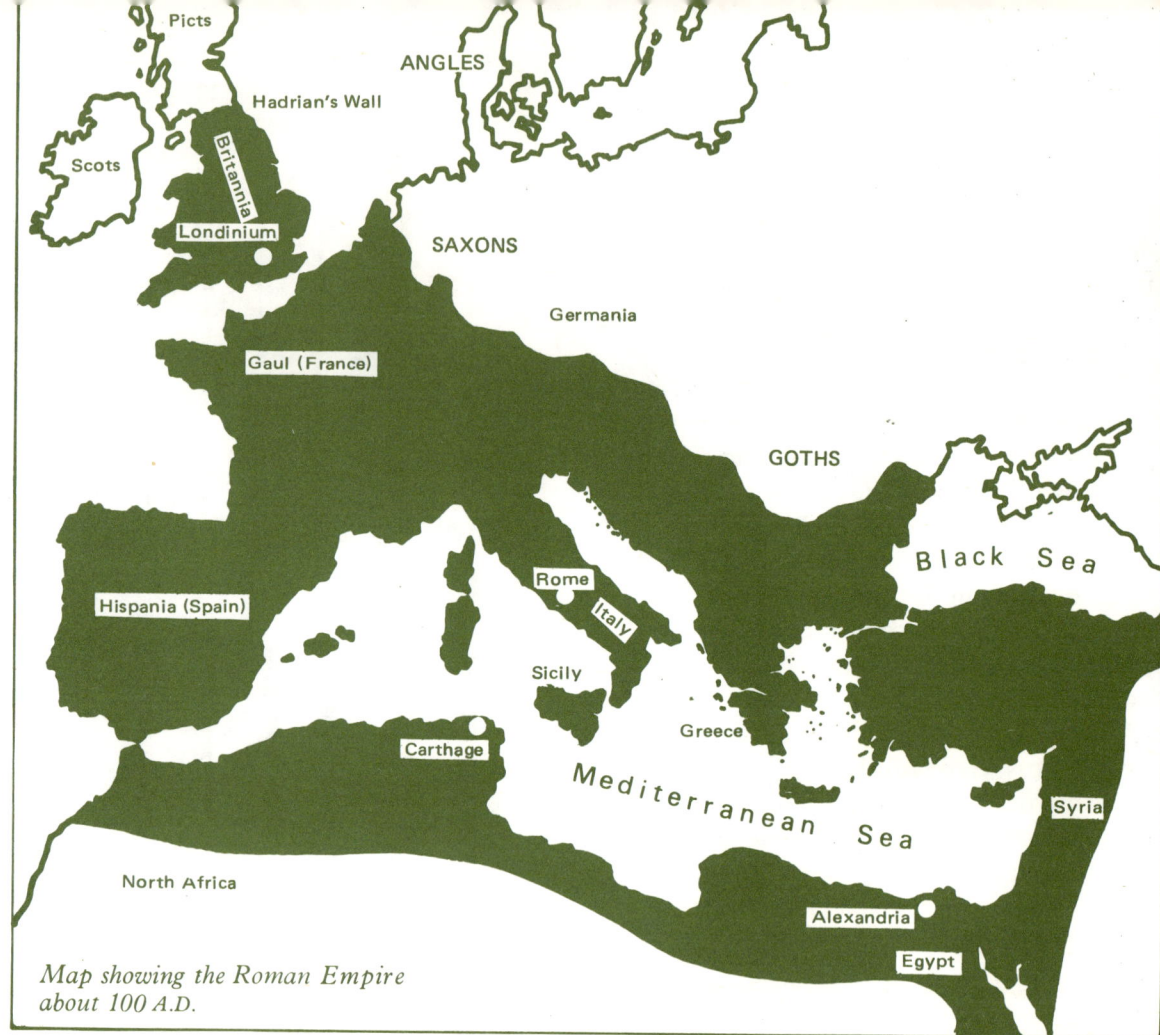

Map showing the Roman Empire about 100 A.D.

The Romans

The Romans became the most powerful people in the Mediterranean area after the Greeks. They were very interested in the Greek way of life—their buildings, their religion, their sports, their pottery and their literature. The Romans first came into contact with the Greeks when colonists settled in southern Italy about 500 B.C. Then in 146 B.C. part of Greece became a province of the Roman Empire. By 27 B.C., when Augustus became the first of the Roman Emperors, the Romans were in firm control not only of Greece but also of the Greek-speaking lands around the Mediterranean.

Although the Romans were attracted by Greek ideas they did not copy them blindly. Perhaps they were more practical and down to earth than the Greeks. Certainly many Romans seem to have distrusted ideas and theories which could not be put to a useful purpose. Strabo, a Greek geographer, tried to sum up the difference between the Greeks and Romans when he said:

The Greeks are famous for their cities and in this they aimed at beauty . . . The Romans excelled in those things which the Greeks took little interest in such as the building of roads, aqueducts and sewers.

(*Geography* Book 5)

This is of course an exaggeration. Perhaps it would be best to say that the Romans had a gift for taking the ideas of other people and putting them to practical use. For example, the Romans were interested in Greek ideas about geometry and mathematics because these subjects helped their engineers and architects to devise new methods of building, especially the construction of domes and arches. Cicero, a Roman writer and orator, made the following comment on Greek and Roman attitudes to science:

The Greeks held the geometer in the highest honour, and, to them, no one came before mathematicians. But we Romans have established as the limit of this art, its usefulness in measuring and reckoning. The Romans have always shown more wisdom than the Greeks in all their inventions, or else improved what they took over from them, such things at least as they thought worthy of serious attention.

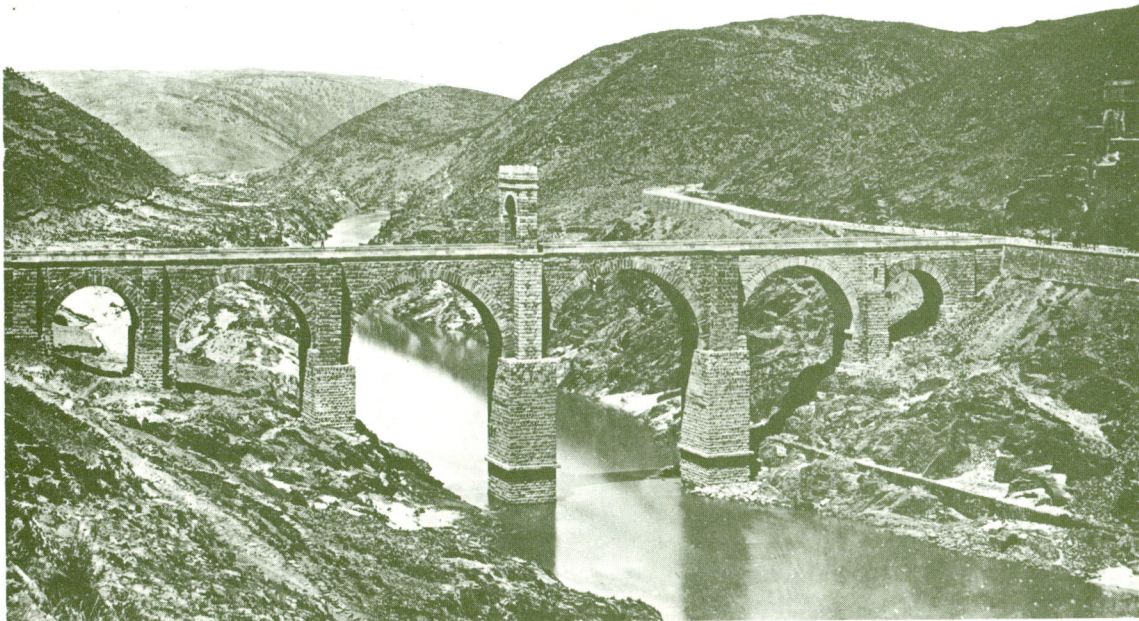

The bridge across the Tagus at Alcantara in Spain built by the Romans in 106 A.D. The central arches are almost 28 metres in diameter

Roman medicine

The Romans were also practical and down to earth in their attitude to medicine and disease. In early times the Romans had no separate medical profession. They believed that each *pater familias* (or head of the household) knew enough about herbs and medicine to treat the illnesses of his own wife, children, slaves and animals. Pliny, a Roman writer, has described some of the remedies they used. Some of these had a sound basis of common sense:

Unwashed wool supplies very many remedies . . . It is applied . . . with honey to old sores. Wounds it heals if dipped in wine or vinegar . . . Yolks of eggs . . . are taken for dysentery with the ash of their shells, poppy juice and wine. It is recommended to bathe the eyes with a decoction of the liver and to apply the marrow to those that are painful or swollen.

(*Natural History* Book 29, chapters 9, 11, 38)

Later, however, as the Roman Empire grew, many Greek doctors came to Rome and Italy. It is not easy to tell exactly what the Romans thought about these Greek doctors. John Scarborough, a recent historian of Roman medicine, has made the following comments on this subject:

At first Hellenistic [Greek or Greek speaking] physicians came to Rome through the purchase of prisoners of war, particularly during the period of Roman expansion in the Hellenistic east to 146 B.C.

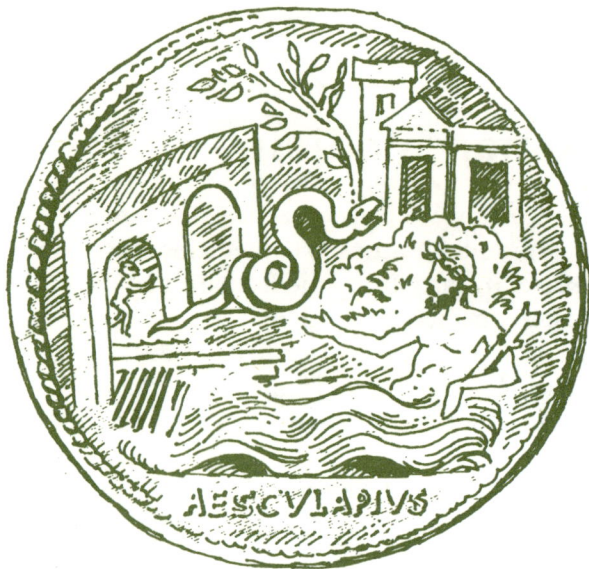

A bronze medallion of Antoninus Pius (138–161 A.D.) showing Father Tiber (Rome's river) welcoming the god Asclepios in the form of a snake. After an outbreak of plague in Rome in 295 B.C. the Romans decided to build a temple to Asclepios on the island in the Tiber. They had heard of the success of Asclepeia in Greece and hoped the Greek god of medicine might be of some use and help to the citizens of Rome

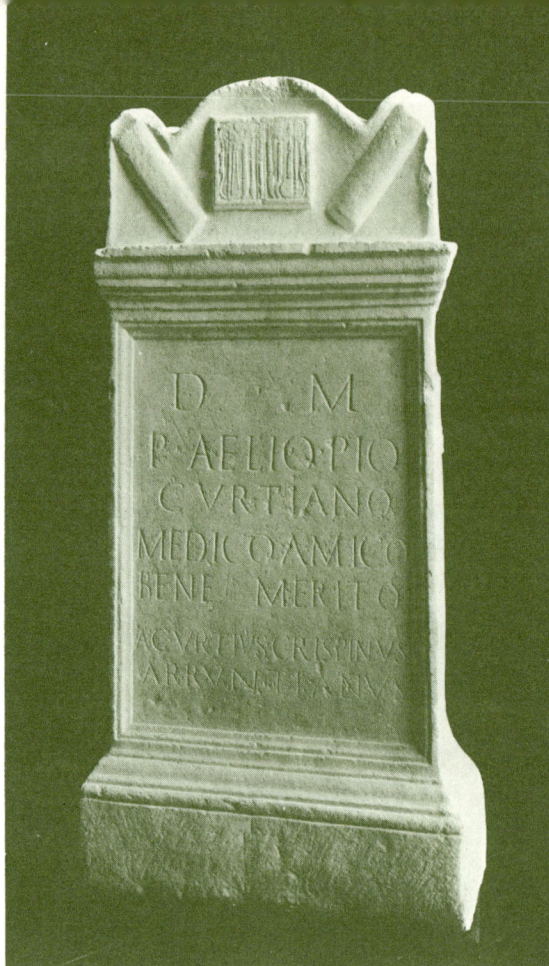

This Roman marble funerary inscription is dedicated to Publius Aelius Pius Curtianus, the freedman or slave doctor of Curtius Crispinus Arruntianus (second century A.D.). At the top is carved a likeness of an open instrument case

Noble Romans who could afford to purchase these highly educated individuals found they made valuable additions to their households and they functioned as personal doctors in the homes of the aristocrats. Many of the slave physicians later obtained their freedom and set up practices of their own in Rome and were joined by numbers of Greek doctors who came to Rome on their own after 200 B.C. Initially the Romans received them warmly, sometimes providing them with shops from which to conduct their practice. Soon, however, the Romans became wary of them with a widespread mistrust.

(*Greek Medicine*, Thames & Hudson 1969, p. 110)

Pliny was one of the Roman writers who seems not to have trusted Greek physicians:

I pass over many famous physicians men like Cassius, Calpetanus, Arruntius and Rubrius. 250 000 sesterces were their annual incomes from the emperors. When Nero was emperor people rushed to Thessalus who swept away all previous ideas. No actor, no driver of a three horse chariot was attended by greater crowds than Thessalus when he walked around in public. Next came Crinas of Massilia [who] regulated the diets of patients by the motions of the stars according to the almanacs of the astronomers . . . Horoscopes

There is no doubt that all these physicians in their hunt for popularity by means of some new idea, did not hesitate to buy it with our lives. Hence those wretched quarrelsome consultations at the bedside of the patients. Hence too that gloomy inscription on monuments 'It was the crowd of physicians which killed me'.

Medicine changes every day and we are swept along on the puffs of the clever brains of the Greeks . . . As if thousands of people do not live without physicians—though not of course, without medicine.

It was not medicine that our forefathers condemned but the medical profession. Our forefathers refused to pay fees to profiteers in order to save their lives. Of all the Greek arts, it is only medicine which we serious Romans have not yet practised.

(*Natural History* Book 29, chapter 8)

Many other Roman writers also seem to have been suspicious of Greek doctors. Yet at the same time some Greek doctors seem to have been very popular. How can we explain this?

John Scarborough, the historian, may

have provided a clue when he wrote that:

Despite the public hue about the poor performance of physicians in the Roman Empire, the best doctors commanded great prestige as they made their rounds and treated their patients.

Perhaps it was the doctors who were not so skilful that Pliny and the other writers were criticising. Perhaps many ordinary people were suspicious of Greek doctors simply because they were foreigners. Others may have been wary of the conflicting medical theories of the Greek doctors. Perhaps the most practical of the Romans simply recognised that there was a limit to what even the best doctors could do when someone was very ill.

Whatever the attitude of ordinary people to Greek doctors, many wealthy Romans seem to have welcomed both Greek doctors and their remedies when they thought them useful.

The Romans and public health

"We must pray for a healthy mind in a healthy body."

The Greek idea which most influenced the Romans was the importance of staying healthy. To the Romans it seemed so much more practical to spend time keeping fit than to spend money on doctors for the sick.

"We must pray for a healthy mind in a healthy body" wrote Juvenal, a Roman poet. Another Roman, Celsus, wrote in his book on medicine that:

A person should put aside some part of the day for the care of his body. He should always make sure that he gets enough exercise especially before a meal.

The forerunners of the Romans

The Romans also came to believe that diseases had natural causes, and that the main dangers to health were bad water and sewage. They were not the first people to realise this. Many rich people in Ancient Egypt had running water or latrines in their homes and the Jews in Old Testament times were very careful about their personal cleanliness.

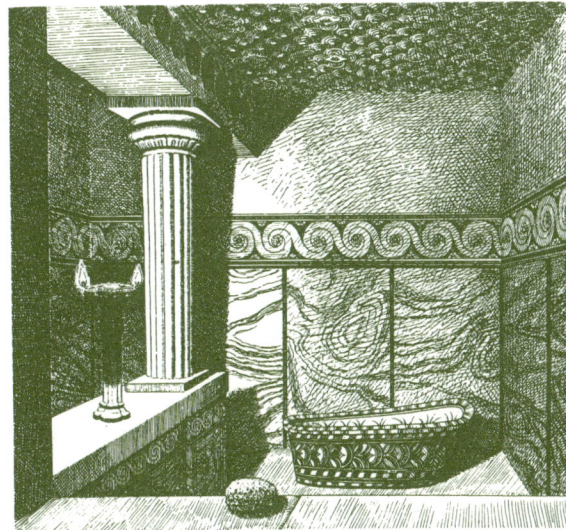

Archaeologists have also unearthed an elaborate system of water supply and drainage in ruined palaces on the island of Crete. They believe that these palaces were inhabited by people between 1900–1400 B.C. Then around 1400 B.C. Crete was devastated by earthquakes and volcanic eruptions which destroyed the palaces and cities, burying them beneath tonnes of ash and lava. They remained hidden and unknown for the next 3300 years. The Romans were forced to find their own answers to problems which Minoan sanitary engineers had already solved. The destruction of the Cretan palaces shows how chance and accidents can prevent change and development in medicine.

The Romans were important because they went much further than any other people in the ancient world. In the same way that they wanted efficient government and just laws for all Roman citizens, rich and poor alike, so the Romans also wanted clean water and good drainage for people throughout their Empire. In other words the Romans were the first people to plan and carry out a programme of public health on a large scale.

The siting of settlements

The Romans believed that it was important to build their settlements—their cities, villas, villages and army forts—in healthy places.

Reconstruction of the Queen's bathroom in the palace at Knossos, Crete

Many Romans wrote warnings about the kind of sites which were unsuitable for human habitation. Marcus Varro in his book on country life wrote:

When building a house or farm especial care should be taken to place it at the foot of a wooded hill where it is exposed to health-giving winds. Care should be taken when there are swamps in the neighbourhood, because certain tiny creatures which cannot be seen by the eyes breed there. These float through the air and enter the body through the mouth and nose and cause serious diseases.

(*Country Life* Book 1, chapter 12)

Columella mentioned similar dangers in his book on country life:

There should be no marshes near buildings, for marshes give off poisonous vapours during the hot period of the summer. At this time, they give birth to animals with mischief-making stings which fly at us in thick swarms.

(*Country Matters* Book 1, chapter 5)

It must have been known from ancient times that mosquitoes and malaria were associated with the same swamps. At first the Romans built a temple to Febris, the goddess of Fever, in the hope of winning her goodwill. Later they took more practical steps and began to drain the marshes from which the malaria arose; for instance, in 398 B.C. an outlet from the Alban Lake was made. Julius Caesar drained the Codetan

The mosquito, the carrier of malaria

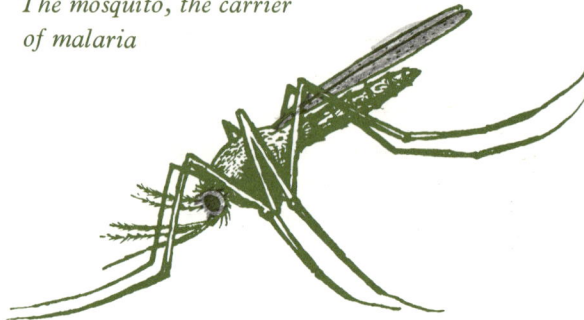

Map showing the site of the Roman settlement of Aquae Sulis (Bath) built where the hot mineral springs burst through the ground. The Romans soon discovered the medicinal qualities of the water and built baths above the spring

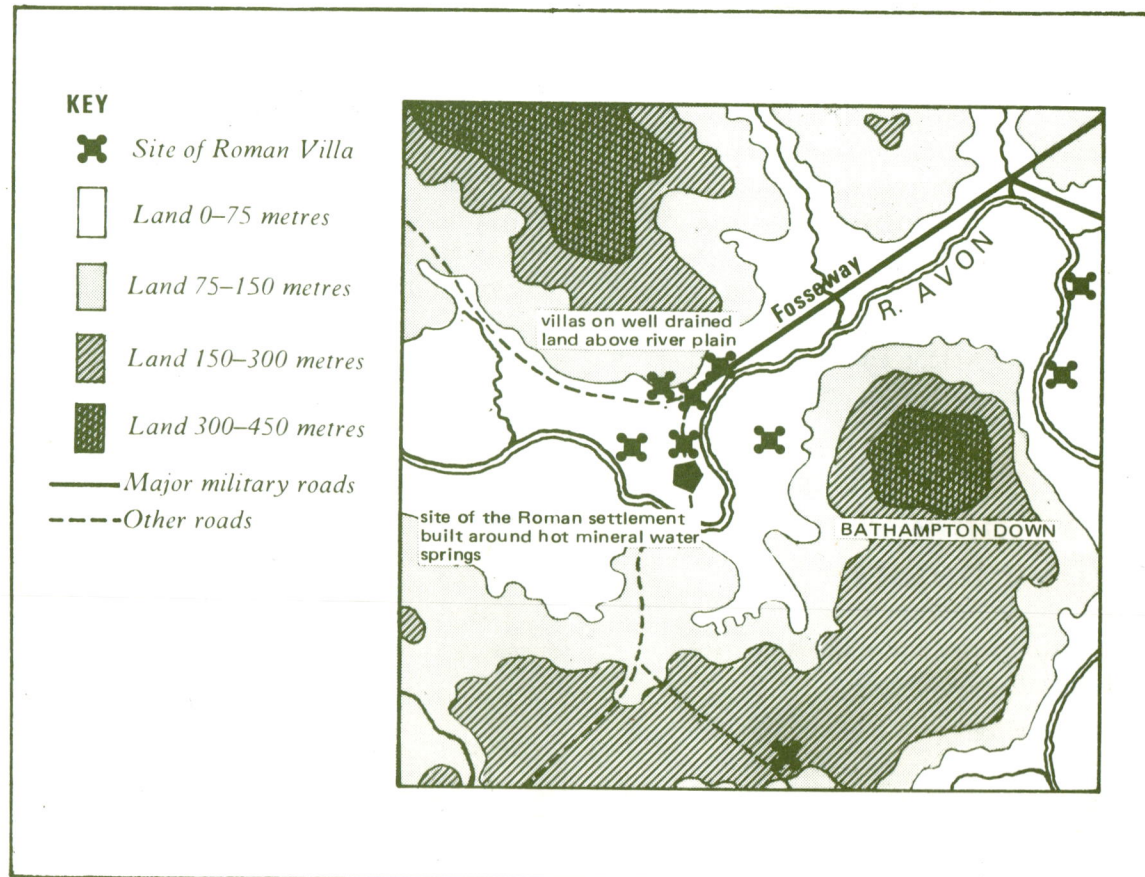

KEY

- ✚ Site of Roman Villa
- Land 0–75 metres
- Land 75–150 metres
- Land 150–300 metres
- Land 300–450 metres
- —— Major military roads
- ---- Other roads

villas on well drained land above river plain

Fosseway

R. AVON

site of the Roman settlement built around hot mineral water springs

BATHAMPTON DOWN

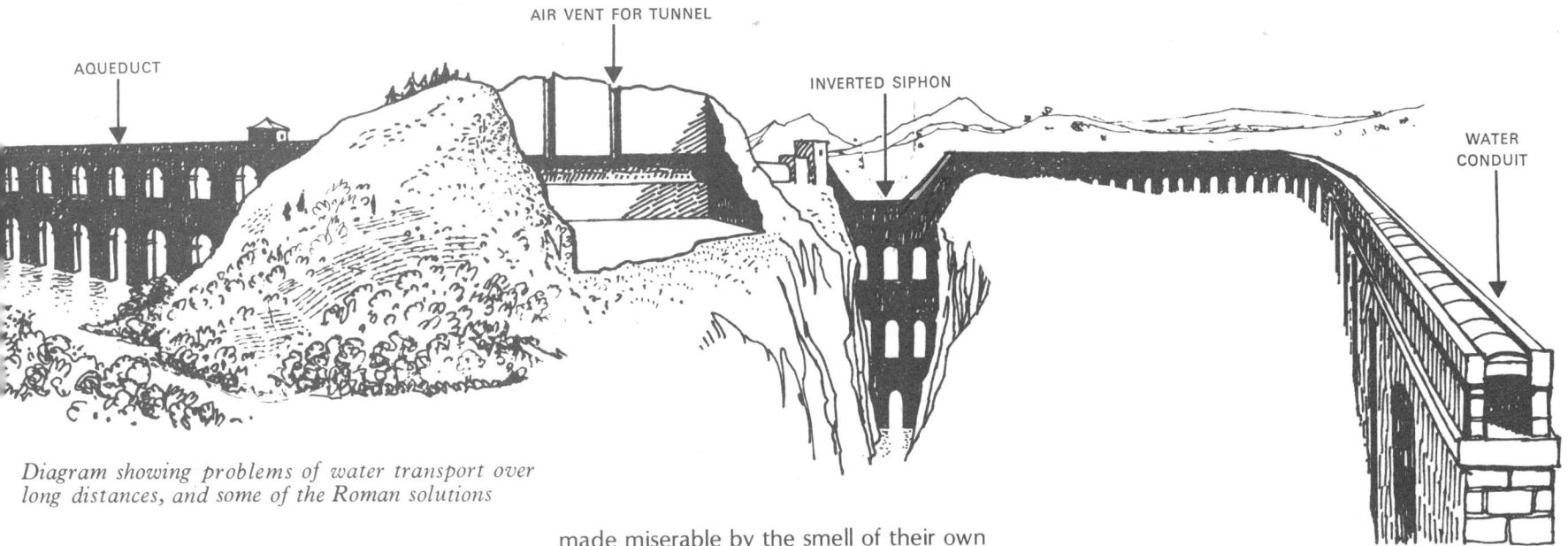

Labels on diagram:
AQUEDUCT
AIR VENT FOR TUNNEL
INVERTED SIPHON
WATER CONDUIT

Diagram showing problems of water transport over long distances, and some of the Roman solutions

Swamp and started a forest in its place.

The health of the soldiers in the Roman Army was always a subject of special concern since they were the men who defended the Empire. Great care was taken to ensure that the soldiers did not fall prey to epidemics in their camps. Vegetius wrote the following advice to Roman army commanders:

I will now give you some ideas about how the army can be kept healthy, by the siting of camps, purity of water, temperature, exercise and medicine. Soldiers must not remain for too long near unhealthy marshes. A soldier who must face the cold without proper clothing is not in a state to have good health or to march. He must not drink swamp water. The generals believe that daily exercise is better for soldiers than physicians. If a group of soldiers is allowed to stay in one place too long in the summer or autumn then they begin to suffer from the effects of polluted water, and are made miserable by the smell of their own excrement. The air becomes unhealthy and they catch diseases. This has to be put right by moving to another camp.

(*Vegetius* Book 3, chapter 2)

Water supplies

The Romans were well aware of the importance of a clean water supply. Vitruvius, a famous Roman architect, mentions this in one of his books on architecture:

We must take great care in searching for springs and, in selecting them, keeping in mind the health of the people. If a spring runs free and open, look carefully at the physique of the people who live nearby before beginning to pipe the water. If their bodies are strong, their complexions fresh, their legs sound and eyes clear then the water is good. If this water is boiled in a bronze cauldron without any sand or mud left in the bottom of the cauldron then the water will be excellent.

(*Vitruvius* Book 8, chapter 3)

The Romans therefore took care to build their forts and towns near good springs, rivers or wells. As these settlements grew, however, they often had to bring water from other springs which were farther away. It was then that Roman engineers were faced with technical difficulties. Their first problem involved water containers, for how were they to transport a huge volume of water from its source to the town or city? Bronze pipes were too expensive over long distances. Lead pipes, when laid underground, were too weak and the Romans did not yet know how to cast large iron pipes which could withstand huge water pressures without breaking. Roman engineers solved the problem by building tunnels of brick or stone known as 'conduits'. Once the water reached the city reservoirs it could then be piped off in small bronze, ceramic or lead pipes.

Their next problem was to make the

water flow along the conduits at a slow and even pace. Since the water could not be pumped the whole way by machine, the Romans built the conduits on a gentle slope all the way from the source of the water to its destination. This presented difficulties when hills or valleys had to be crossed, but the Romans overcame these in ingenious ways, as the diagram indicates, (see p. 41).

When taking conduits across valleys the engineers built them on top of arches of stonework. These looked like bridges and were called *aqueducts*. The height of the aqueducts varied according to the valley. When hills could not be avoided, engineers built tunnels to take the water through. Air vents were made every 240 feet (73 metres) to prevent airlocks and allow for inspection and cleaning. Water was carried across narrow gorges by means of inverted syphons. The conduit was built in the shape of a flat bottomed V. Water flowed down one side and was then forced across and up the other side by atmospheric pressure. The opening on this side had to be slightly lower than that of the first one.

The water supply of Rome

The water supply of Rome, the capital of the Empire, was a masterpiece of engineering. Julius Frontinus was appointed Water Commissioner for Rome in 97 A.D. by the Emperor Nerva. He described the aqueducts of the city which he estimated to bring 222 236 060 gallons (about 1000 million litres) of water a day into Rome.

My job concerns not merely the convenience, but also the health of the city and so this task has always been handled by the most important men in the State.

For 441 years after the foundation of the city, Romans were satisfied to use water from the Tiber and nearby wells or springs. But now 9 aqueducts bring water into the city. When M. Valerius Maximus and P. Decius Mus were consuls, the Appian aqueduct was built. 40 years later the two censors, Marius Curius and Lucius Papirius contracted to build the Old Anio aqueduct with money from the war booty. Two water commissioners were appointed to take charge of this. In order to bring the water into the city on a gentle slope the conduit had to be made 43 000 paces long.

127 years later the Senate commissioned Marcius the Praetor to repair the Appian and the Old Anio aqueducts because they were becoming old and leaky and also

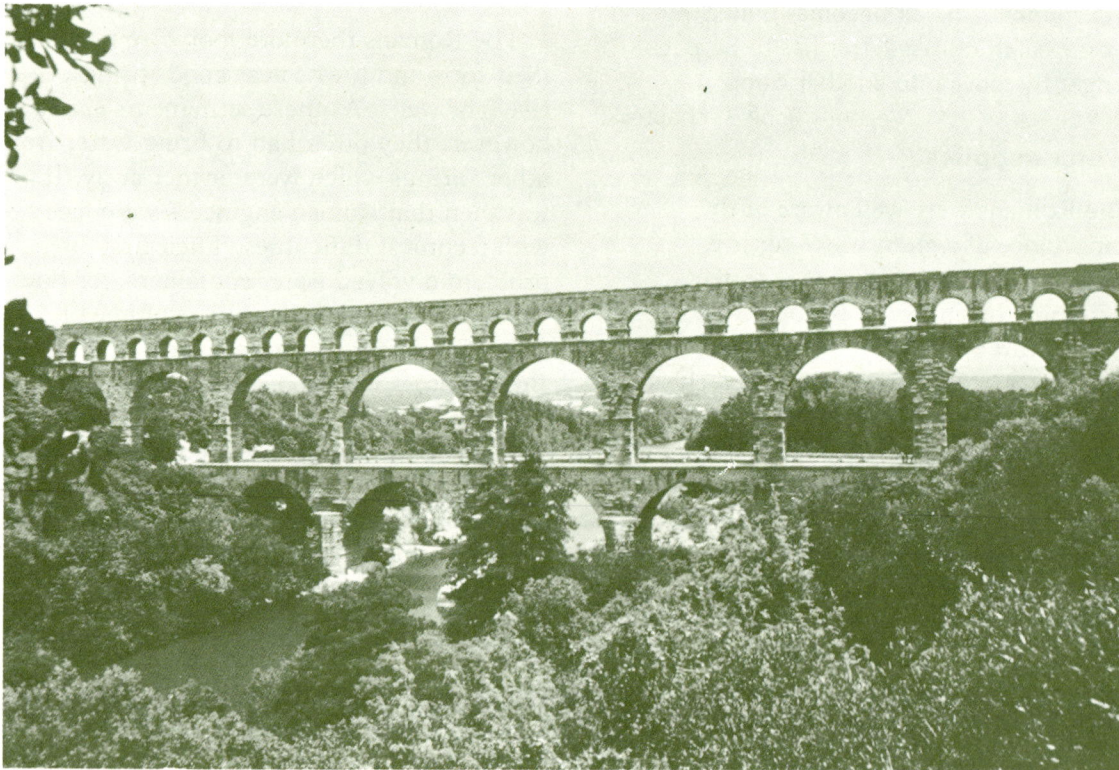

Pont du Gard Roman aqueduct, Nîmes, southern France

some people were illegally channelling off water from them.

The new Anio aqueduct is taken from the river which is muddy and discoloured because of the ploughed fields on either side. Because of this a special filter tank was placed at the beginning of the aqueduct where the soil could settle and the water clarify before going along the channel. Six other aqueducts have filter tanks about 7 miles [11 kilometres] outside the city on the Latin Way.

The aqueducts reach the city at different levels so that some deliver water to the high ground and some to the lower ground. Compare such important engineering works carrying so much water with the idle pyramids and the useless though famous buildings of the Greeks!

(*The Aqueducts of Rome* Prologue and Book 1)

Strabo, a Greek geographer, marvelled at the water supply when he visited Rome in the first century B.C.:

Water is brought into the city through aqueducts in such quantities that it is like a river flowing through the city. Almost every house has cisterns and water pipes and fountains.

(*Geography* Book 5)

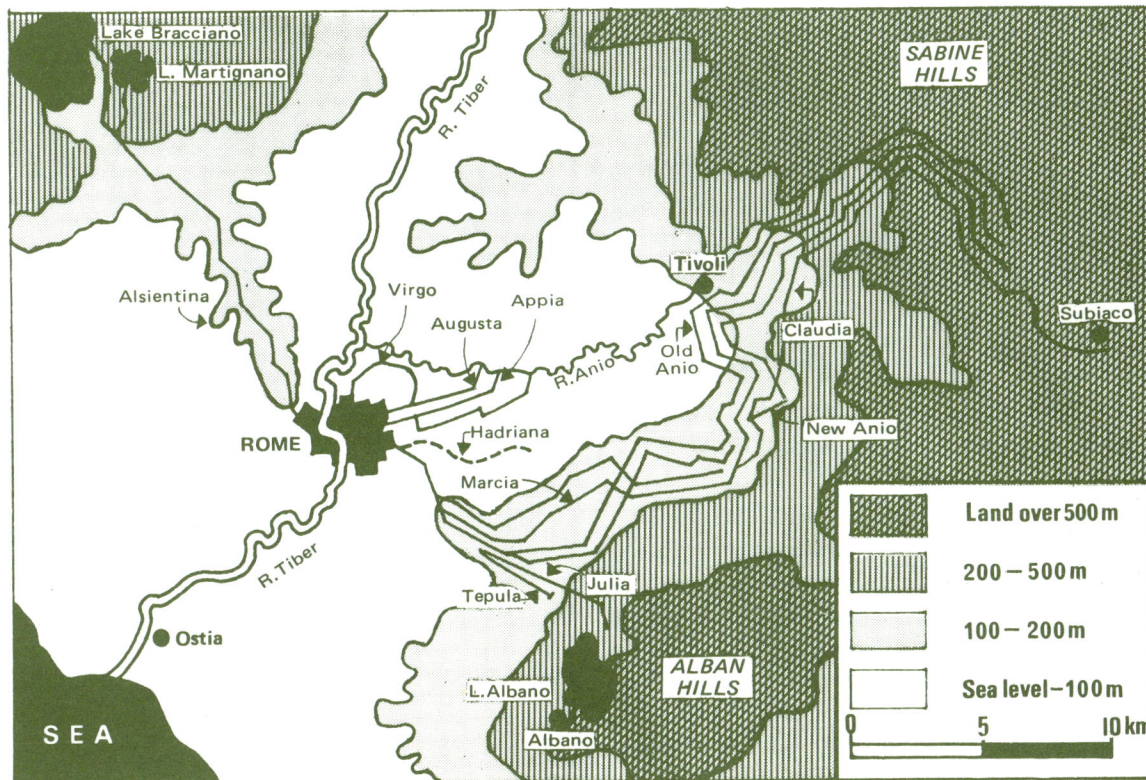

Map showing the routes of the Roman aqueducts

At the Emperor's disposal	17·1%
To private persons (houses and industries)	38·6%
Public supplies:	
(a) 19 military barracks	2·9%
(b) 95 official buildings	24·1%
(c) 39 public buildings, baths and theatres	3·9%
(d) 591 cisterns and fountains	13·4%
TOTAL	100·0%

Distribution figures for the water supply of Rome (according to Frontinus)

43

The public baths

The Romans also believed in the importance of personal cleanliness and realised that this too was essential for good health. They were, perhaps, introduced to the idea by the Greeks, but once the Romans had become convinced of its usefulness they set about making daily bathing a possibility for all citizens, rich and poor alike. Wherever the Romans settled, in town or fort throughout their Empire, they built public baths. Opening hours were usually from 1 p.m. to dusk and the entrance fee was minimal—usually about a *quadrans* (one-sixteenth of 1p!).

By 50 A.D., when Seneca was writing his famous letters, the Romans were obviously spending vast amounts of money on their public baths. Here are some of Seneca's comments on them:

In the early days there were few baths. Bathers of those days did not have fresh water poured over them. They did not worry about the water being pure when they knew they were only going to make it dirty! Nevertheless, the aediles used to inspect these baths and make sure that they were kept clean and warm enough for comfort and health.

But who in these days could bear to bathe in such a fashion! We think ourselves poor if our walls are not covered with huge mirrors, if our ceilings are not buried in glass and our swimming pools lined with marble, and if the water does not pour from silver

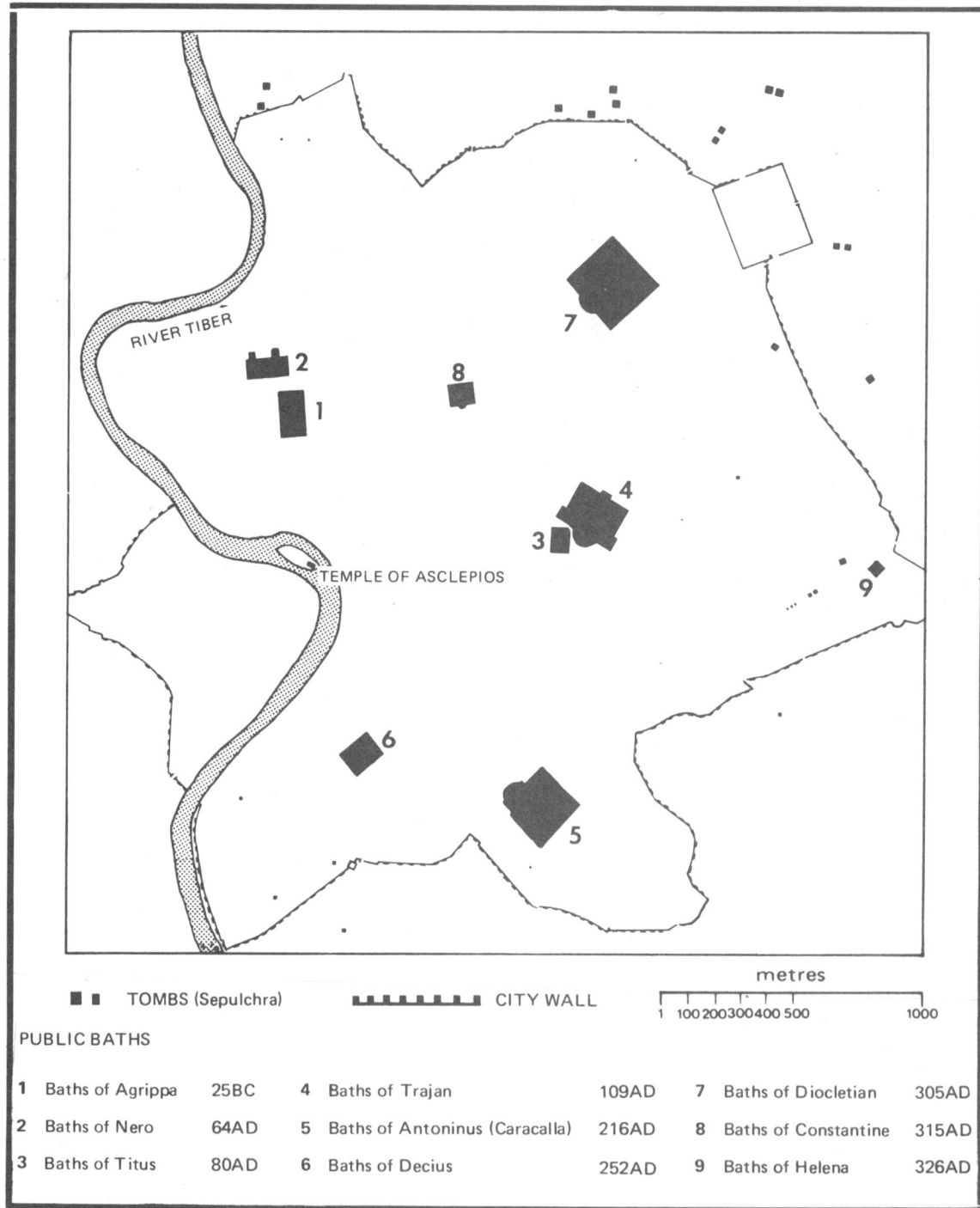

RIVER TIBER

TEMPLE OF ASCLEPIOS

metres

■ ■ TOMBS (Sepulchra)	▪▪▪▪▪▪▪ CITY WALL	1 100 200 300 400 500 1000

PUBLIC BATHS

1	Baths of Agrippa	25BC	4	Baths of Trajan	109AD	7	Baths of Diocletian	305AD
2	Baths of Nero	64AD	5	Baths of Antoninus (Caracalla)	216AD	8	Baths of Constantine	315AD
3	Baths of Titus	80AD	6	Baths of Decius	252AD	9	Baths of Helena	326AD

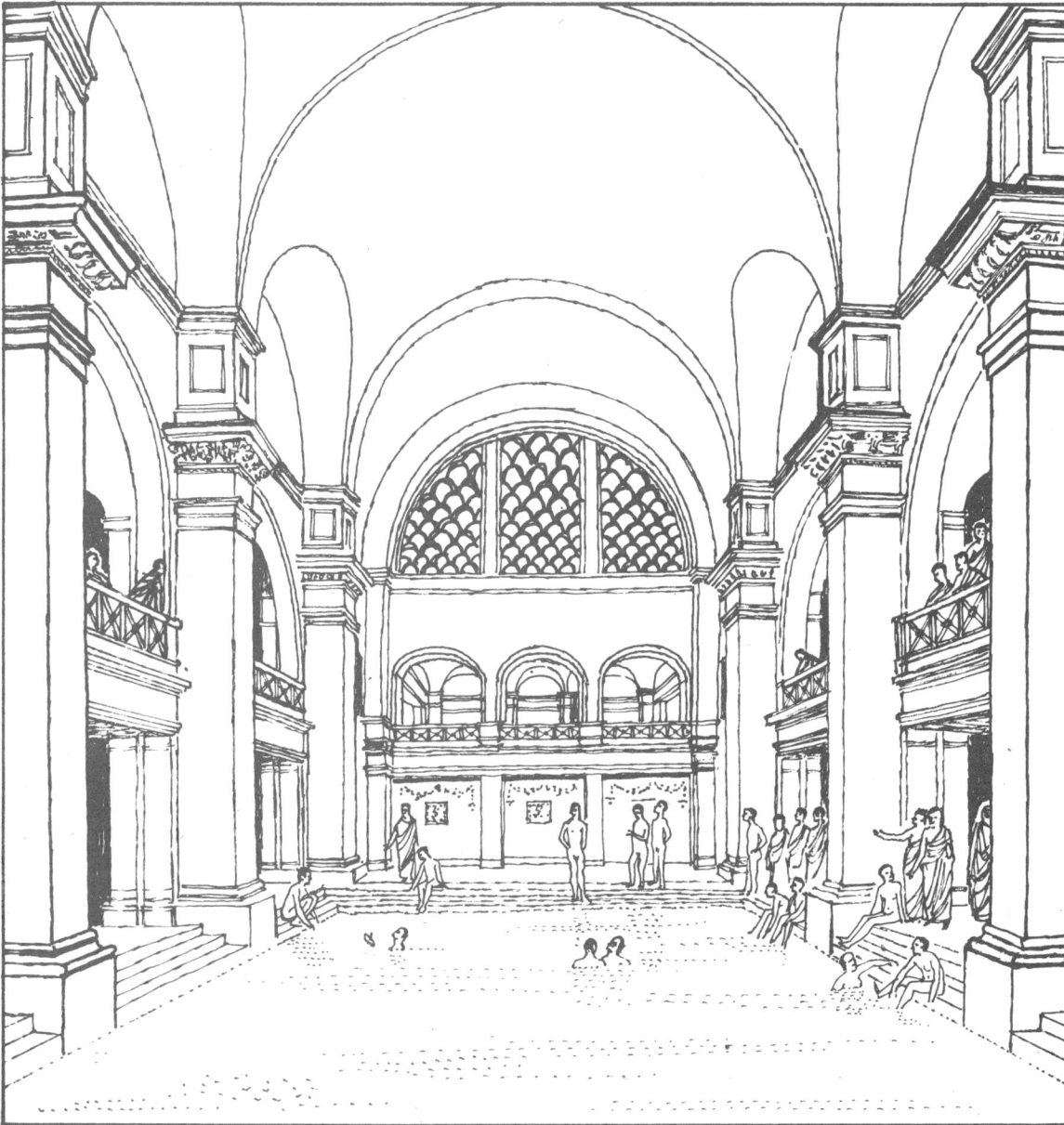

spouts! And I am talking only about the baths of the common people! What about the baths of the freedmen—all the statues, all the masses of water tumbling from level to level.

(Letter LXXX)

The Romans believed that bathing was as good for the sick as it was essential for the healthy. Celsus, a Roman writer, recommended a visit to the baths for any person with "a weak part of the body":

I have next to speak of those who have some weak part of the body. If a man goes to the baths he should first stay wrapped up and sweat for a while in the tepidarium. Then he should be anointed with oil. Next he should go into the caldarium. After a further sweat he should not go as usual into the hot bath but should have a shower from the head downwards first with hot then tepid, and finally cold water. This should be poured longest on his head. After this he should be rubbed down for a while and finally wiped and oiled. Nothing is so good for the head as cold water.

(Medical Matters Book 1, chapter 4)

The great bath at Aquae Sulis (present-day Bath)

45

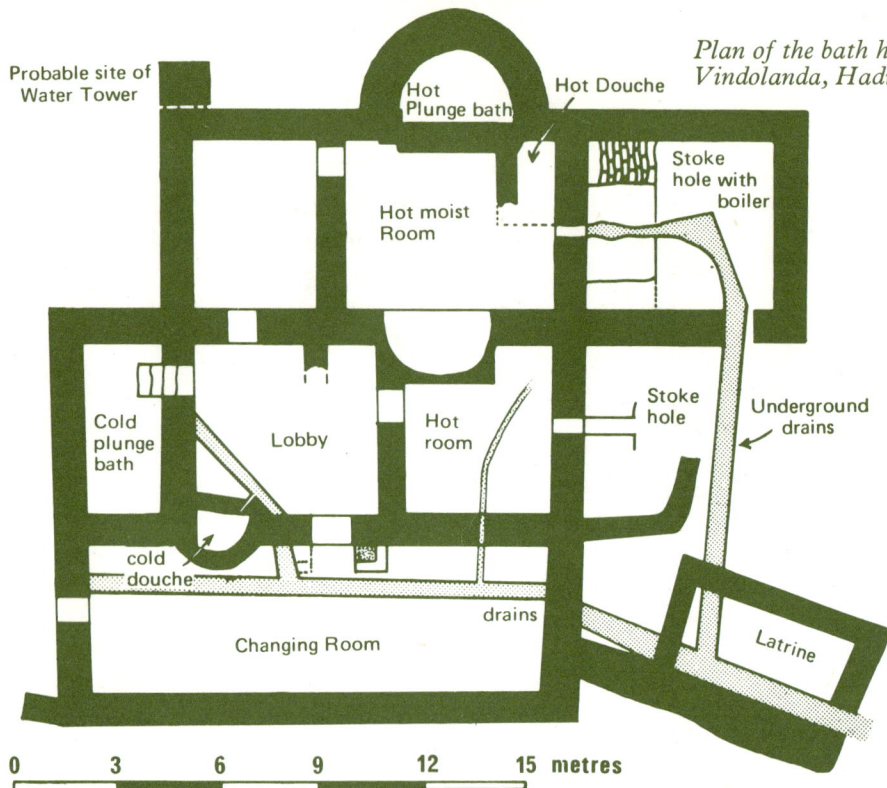

Plan of the bath house at the Roman fort of Vindolanda, Hadrian's wall, Northumberland

Probable site of Water Tower

Hot Plunge bath

Hot Douche

Hot moist Room

Stoke hole with boiler

Cold plunge bath

Lobby

Hot room

Stoke hole

cold douche

Underground drains

drains

Changing Room

Latrine

0 3 6 9 12 15 metres

Drainage and sewage disposal

The Romans' interest in hygiene also led them to build latrines. Latrines were not new. Archaeologists have discovered them in the houses of the rich people in ancient Babylon, Crete and Egypt, but the Romans intended to make these available to *all* their citizens. Public latrines were built in the town streets, in military forts, and at the baths. By 315 A.D. it is estimated that Rome had 144 such latrines flushed by water. Private individuals also installed them in their homes.

The building of baths, fountains and latrines meant that Roman towns and forts

Latrines in Housesteads Roman Fort, Hadrian's wall, Northumberland. Wooden seats would have covered the drains on the left and right of the block

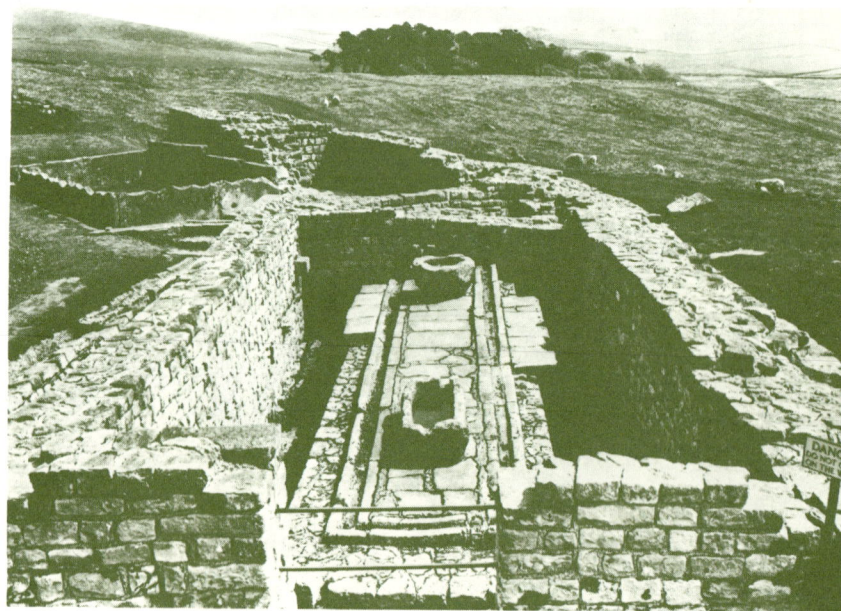

Diagram to show how the rooms of the baths were

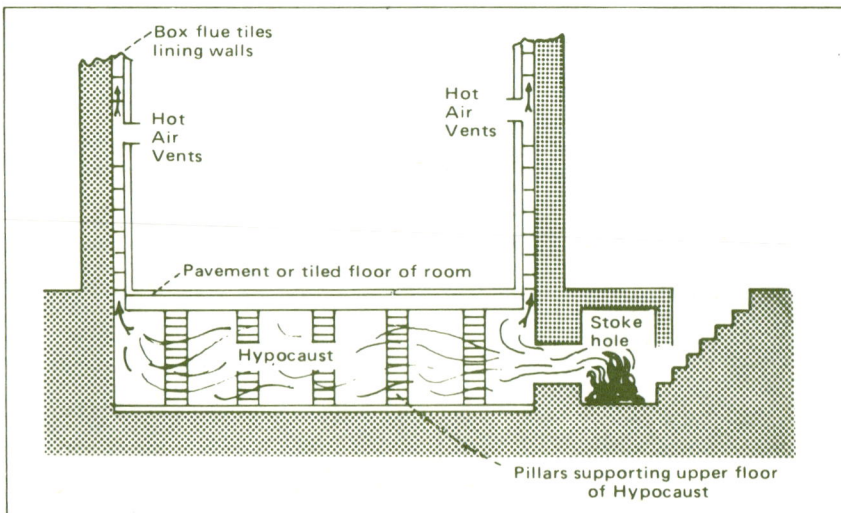

Box flue tiles lining walls

Hot Air Vents

Hot Air Vents

Pavement or tiled floor of room

Hypocaust

Stoke hole

Pillars supporting upper floor of Hypocaust

46

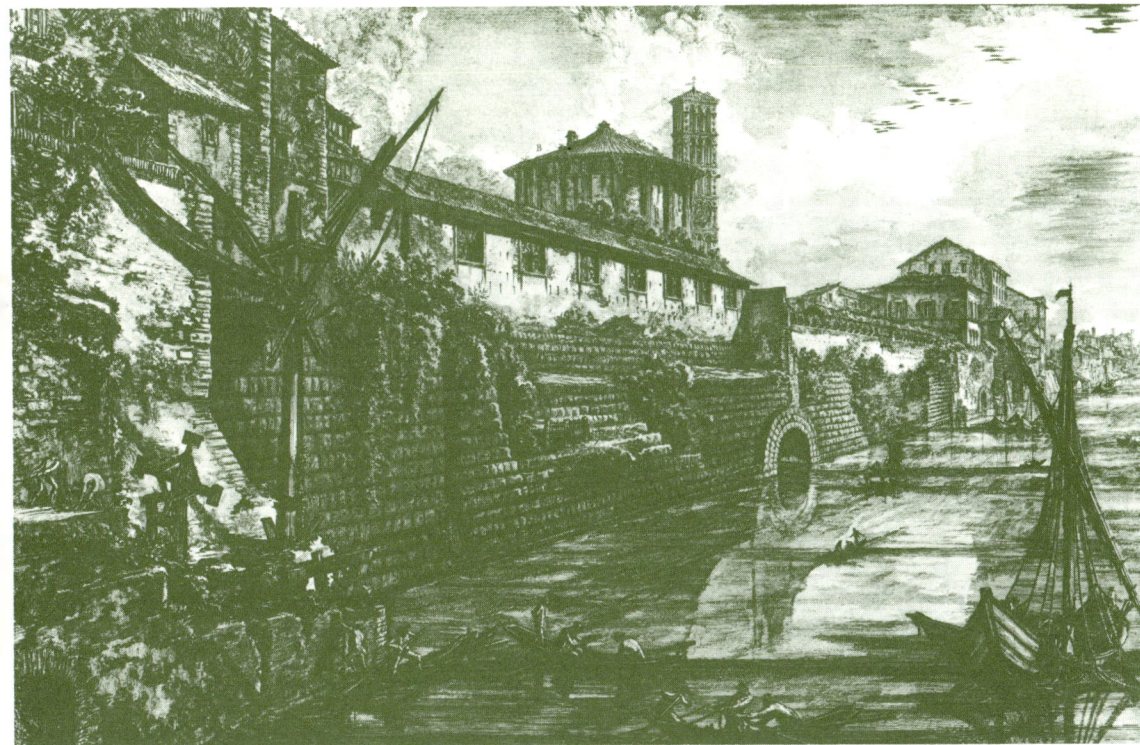

Outlet into the River Tiber of the 'Cloaca Maxima', the great sewer of Rome

Public latrines at the Hadrianic Baths at Leptis Magna, North Africa

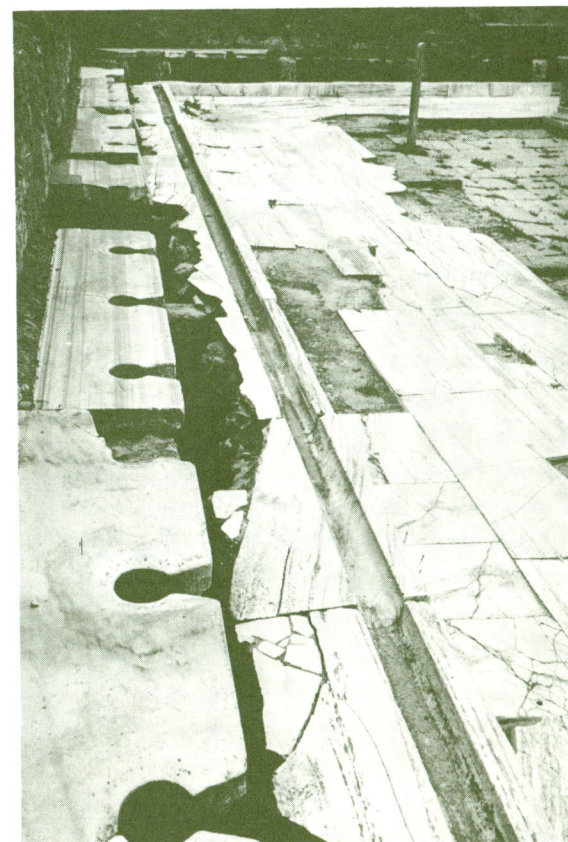

needed an efficient drainage system. Pliny, a Roman writer, described the drainage system of Rome:

Old men still admire the city sewers, the greatest achievement of all. They were built 700 years ago in the days of Tarquinius Priscus and they are still undamaged. Tarquinius is said to have made the tunnels large enough for a waggon load of hay to pass through. Hills were tunnelled and Rome became like a hanging city. When Marcus Agrippa became aedile in 33 B.C. he travelled on a tour of inspection under the city in a boat. There are 7 rivers made to flow in 7 tunnels under the city, these finally run into one great sewer. These rivers rush through like mountain streams and, swollen by the rain water, they sweep away all the sewage. The bottom and sides of the sewers take a real hammering!

(*Natural History* Book 36, chapter 105)

Military hospitals

Concern for the health of the army also led the Romans to develop military hospitals, especially on the frontiers of their Empire. Examples of such hospitals have been discovered in Switzerland, Germany and North Africa as well as in Britain.

The hospitals were not remarkable for the treatment they gave to the wounded—it was fairly rudimentary. The soldiers were tended by *medici* (medical officers) who were probably, in fact, ordinary soldiers who had shown an aptitude for such work and had acquired skill in dealing with wounds over a number of years. The army commander usually had a personal surgeon and though he may have helped on occasions, his duties were really to travel with the commander and not to remain behind near the hospital.

It was the drainage and sanitation systems of the hospitals which made them a model for the future. At Inchtuthil in Scotland, archaeologists have uncovered the outlines of a large military hospital with a superb drainage system into one of the camp sewers. A similar one was built at Abergavenny, in Gwent.

Hygiene was obviously considered essential if the wounded were to get back to battle as quickly as possible and were not to succumb to the enemy of disease beforehand.

General plan of the Roman military hospital at Novaesium (near Dusseldorf, modern Germany)

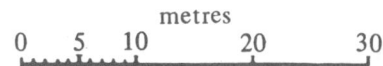

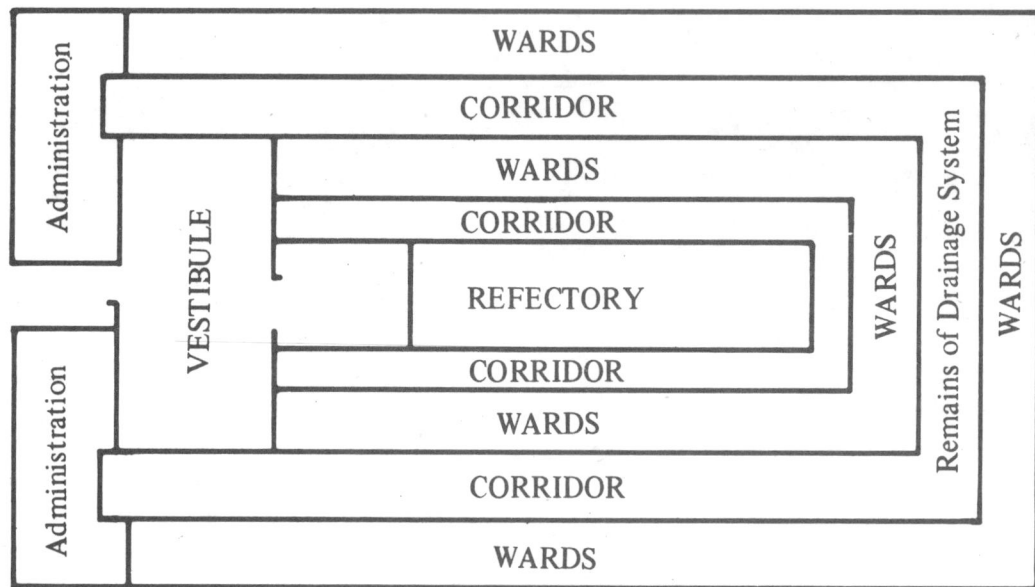

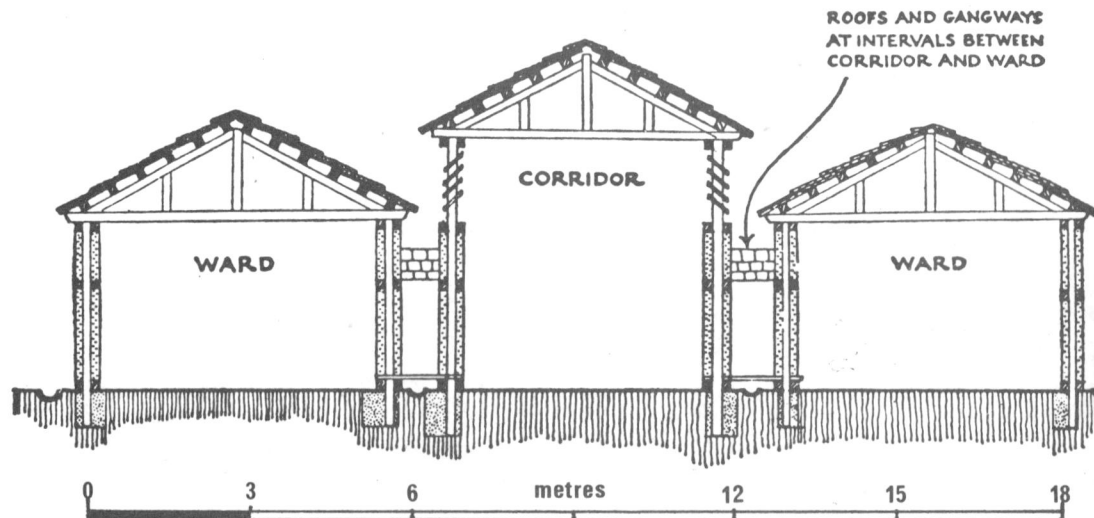

Cross section of part of the Roman Legionary Hospital at Inchtuthil

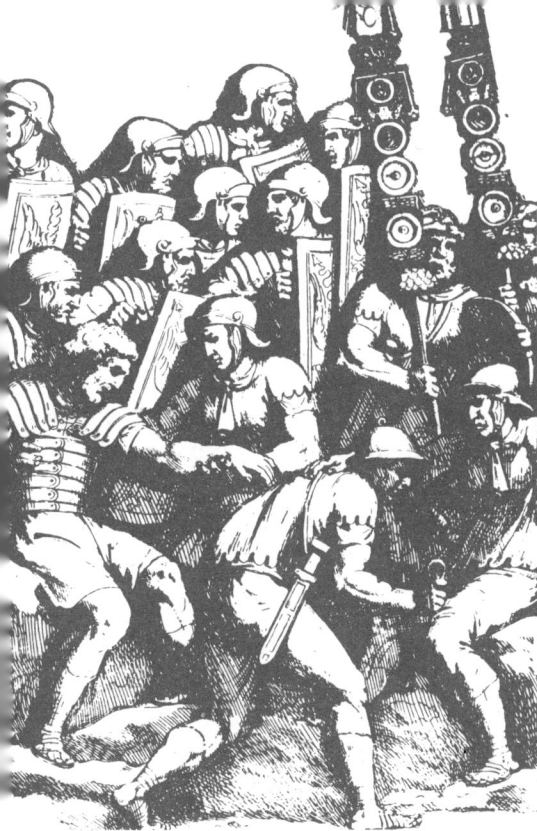

A drawing from a section of Trajan's column in Rome showing two legionary 'medici' at work helping wounded soldiers. Note the similarity in uniform between the soldiers and the 'medici'

Roman public health: some conclusions

The Romans did more than any other people before them to keep the mass of people healthy by helping to prevent those diseases which are caused by polluted water and insanitary conditions. They were justly proud of their achievements, as Frontinus reveals in his book about the aqueducts of Rome:

The result of this care can be seen each day in the improved health of Rome, because of the great number of reservoirs, works, fountains and water basins. The appearance of the city is cleaner and changed and the causes of the unhealthy air, which gave Rome such a bad name amongst the people in the past, are now removed.

(*The Aqueducts of Rome* Book 2, chapter 8)

We must, however, be careful not to assume that the Roman system of water supply and drainage was as effective as

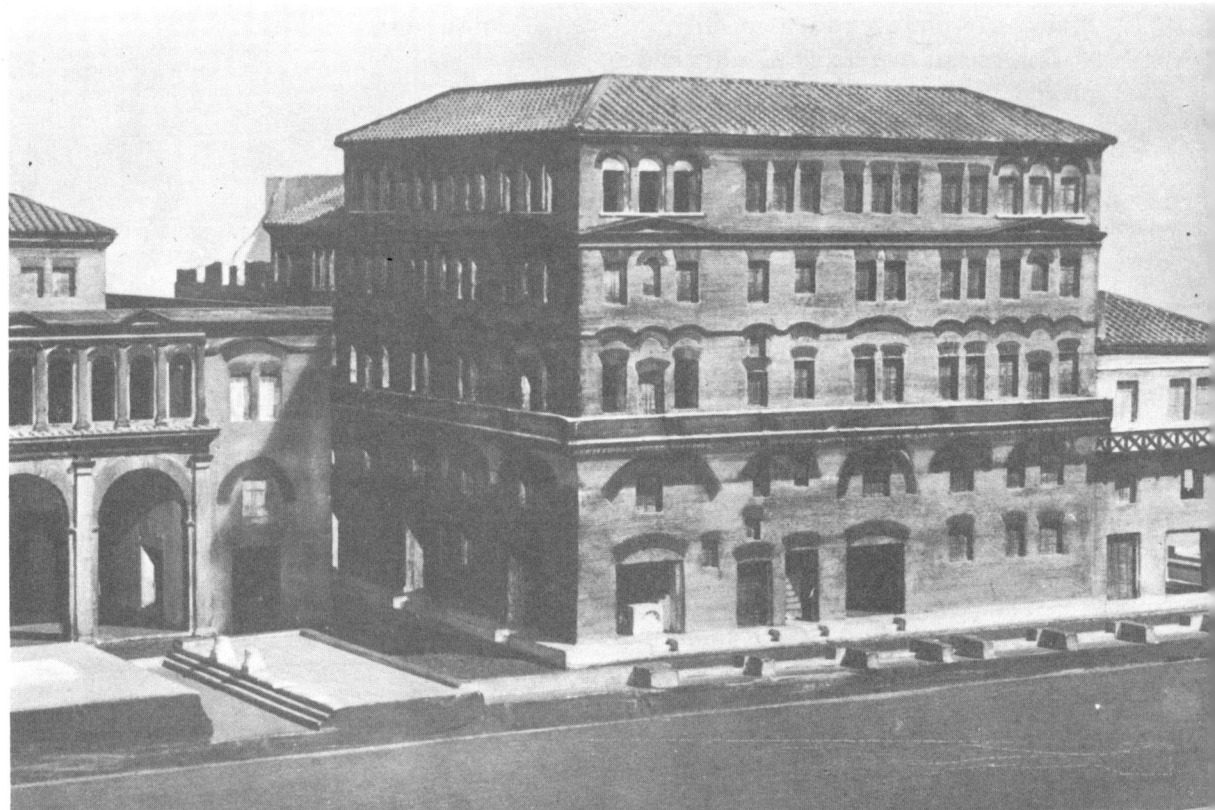

Model reconstruction of a five-storey tenement block at Ostia, near Rome

modern systems. There were some technical problems which even the Romans could not solve.

In particular, they seem to have found it either too difficult or too expensive to install water and sewage pipes in the upstairs rooms of their apartment blocks. Archaeologists excavating apartment blocks in Ostia, Herculaneum and Rome have so far discovered evidence of plumbing and drainage on the ground floors only.

This meant that many families had a problem of waste disposal, and the solution they sometimes adopted, though simple, was also very unhygienic. It certainly caused one Roman writer, Juvenal, to issue a warning to passers-by in the street:

Along your route each open window may be a death trap. So hope and pray, you poor man, that the local housewives drop nothing worse on your head than a bedpan full of slops!

(*Satires* Book 3, lines 269–272)

Despite these technical problems, the Romans had brought about remarkable changes in the lives of ordinary people, even in countries far away from Rome and Italy. Yet two interesting questions about the achievements of the Romans still remain to be considered. First, why did they not continue to develop Greek ideas about the investigation and treatment of disease? Why did they choose instead to concentrate on public health schemes? You have already read some possible reasons earlier in this section. Can you think of any more? Secondly, why were the Romans so successful in spreading their ideas about public health far and wide at a time when communications over long distances were still difficult? What difference did it make that they had *conquered* these countries and were able, in time, to bring a peaceful and orderly life to their inhabitants? Discuss these questions and see what reasons you can suggest.

Greek doctors in the Roman world

Since the Romans showed little interest in the medical theories of Hippocrates and the Greeks, it was left to the Greek doctors who had settled in Italy to pursue scientific methods of observation.

In some aspects of medicine progress was made, especially by the surgeons who,

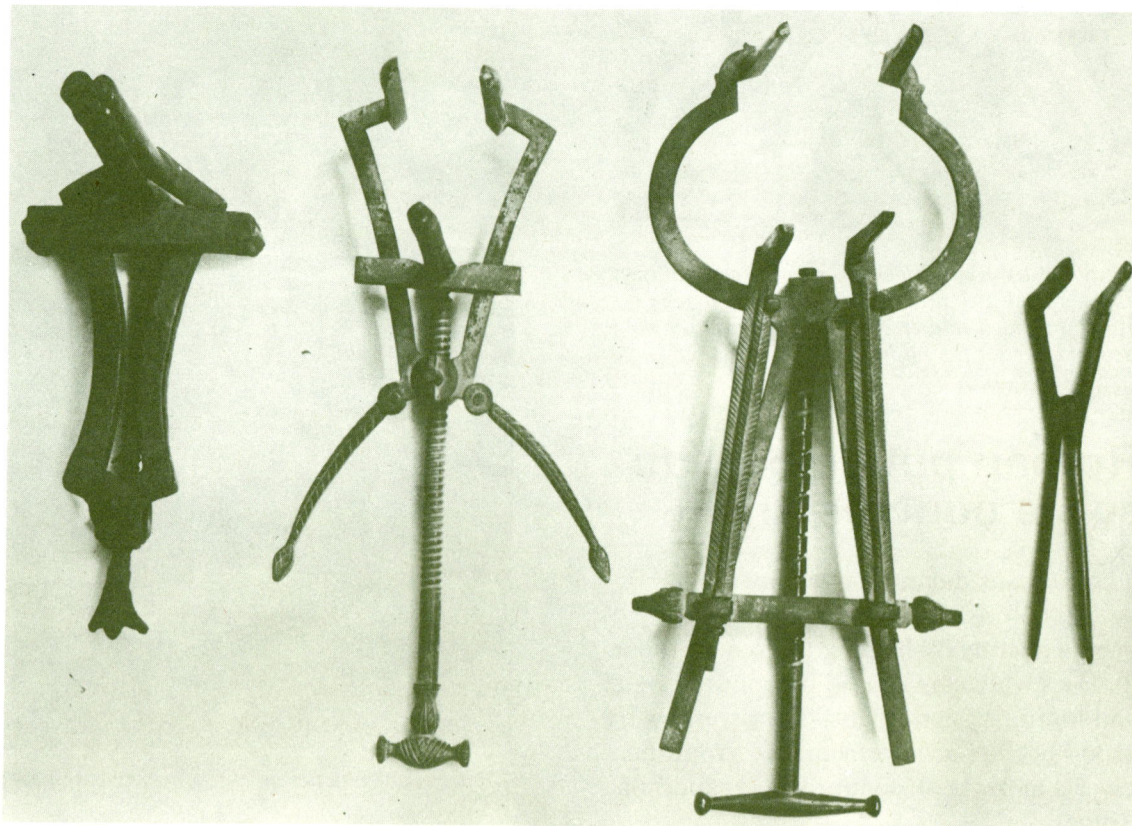

Roman surgical and midwifery instruments

because of the nature of their work, tended to be practical men. New instruments were devised to help the surgeons perform intricate operations, such as the removal of polyps from the nose and goitres from the throat. Plastic surgery was sometimes carried out on the face and mouth.

Dioscorides, a Greek who served as surgeon in Nero's army, collected specimens of herbs from all over the known world as he travelled with the armies. He gathered all this knowledge together in a book about herbs and medicine. In his *Herbarium* Dioscorides described plants and listed all the diseases they could be used to cure. This book became famous and was used by doctors for the next 1600 years.

Unlike the surgeons, Greek physicians made little progress. In fact far from learning new things, too many Greek doctors had not even adopted the fine clinical methods of Hippocrates.

As Pliny's account on page 38 suggests, many Greek doctors became involved in long arguments about diseases and treatments which were no longer based on careful observations, but on untested theories.

It was Claudius Galen, a Greek doctor from Pergamum in Asia Minor, who came to Rome and revived the ideas and methods of Greek doctors in Hippocrates' time.

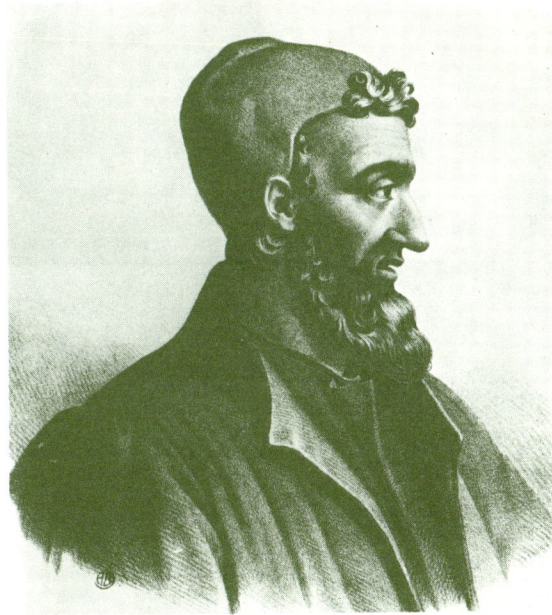

An imaginary portrait of Galen (after a sixteenth-century engraving)

Claudius Galen and his work

Life and background

Galen was born about 131 A.D., the son of Nicon, a wealthy architect. He seems to have inherited the brains of his father and the bad temper of his mother! Galen said of her, "my mother used to bite her maids and was always shouting at my father". Nicon, however, had hopefully given his son a name which means 'peaceable'. It is said that Nicon learned in a dream that his son would be a physician and so he sent Galen to study at the famous medical school at Alexandria in Egypt. When he was twenty-eight years old, Galen became surgeon to a school of gladiators, but in 161 A.D. he went to Rome to seek his fortune. He stayed there for several years,

becoming famous for his experiments and treatments. In 166 A.D. however, he was forced to leave the city—perhaps because of the jealousy of the other doctors. In 168 A.D. he was hastily summoned back to Rome by the Emperors Marcus Aurelius and Verus. Verus died of plague and Galen was given medical charge of Marcus Aurelius' heir, Commodus. At this time he began his medical writing. He died aged about seventy, in 201 A.D.

Galen and the revival of Hippocratic methods

Galen revived the methods used by doctors in Hippocrates' time but which were falling into disuse. He practised Hippocratic methods of clinical observation—examining his patients carefully and noting their symptoms. He also accepted the theory that disease was the result of an imbalance in the four liquids of the body—blood, phlegm, black and yellow bile.

Galen's treatments: the 'use of opposites'

Although he believed, like Hippocrates, in the healing power of nature, Galen went further than Hippocrates in developing treatments to restore the balance of the four humours. He believed in the 'use of opposites'. This involved treatments such as pepper, which would bring heat to a man whose disease was thought to be caused by cold, or cucumber which would cool a man whose illness was thought to be caused by heat. Violent gymnastic exercises were prescribed for weak or convalescent people; singing and breathing exercises for a man with a deformed chest.

Galen and anatomy

In the time of Hippocrates, Greek doctors had recorded little new information about the structure and workings of the body. Galen, however, realised that such knowledge was very important to the physician. He dissected many pigs and apes and studied their bone structure, muscles and nerves in great detail. There is also evidence to suggest that Galen had witnessed and perhaps even carried out human dissection. Galen certainly thought the study of the human body was very important. He always advised his pupils to dissect apes because of their resemblance to humans, as the following extract from one of his books shows:

> Human bones are subjects of study with which you should first become perfectly familiar. You cannot merely read about bones in . . . books . . . but [must] also acquaint yourself with the appearance of each of the bones, by the use of your own eyes, handling each bone by itself . . .
>
> At Alexandria this is very easy, since the physicians in that country accompany their lessons to their students with opportunities for personal inspection [of human bodies]. Hence you must try to get to Alexandria for this reason alone if no other. But if you cannot manage this, it is not impossible to

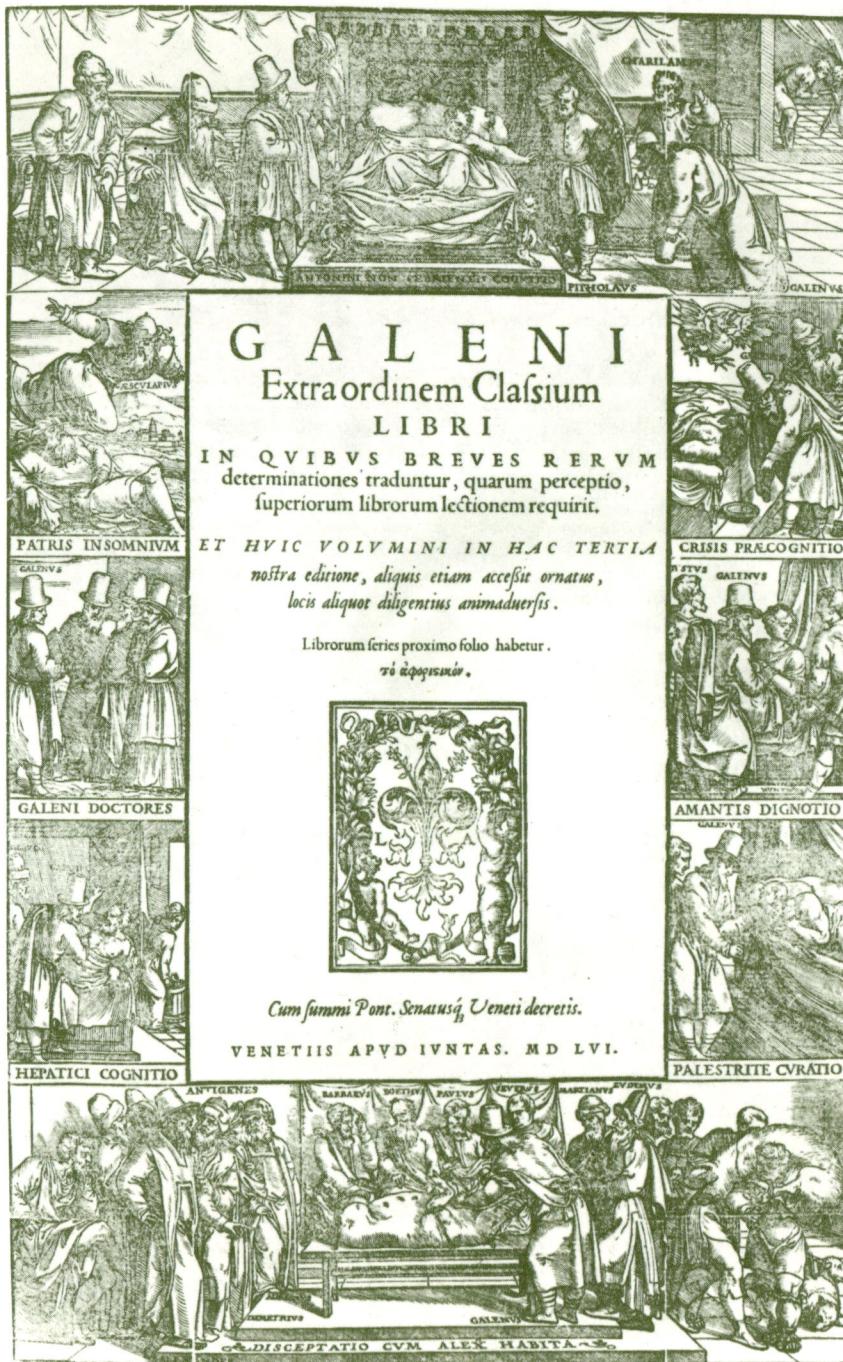

This is the title page from an edition of Galen's collected works. Notice the woodcut at the bottom which depicts Galen's experiments on the nerves of a pig. An enlarged detail is shown on page 53 opposite

obtain a view of human bones. Personally I have often had a chance to do this where tombs or monuments have become broken up. On one occasion a river . . . caused . . . a grave to disintegrate . . . and then carried the corpse away downstream [eventually] . . . depositing it. Here the corpse lay ready for inspection, just as though prepared by a doctor for his pupils' lesson.

Once I also examined the skeleton of a robber lying on a mountain-side a short distance from the road . . . So if you do not have the luck to see anything like this, you can still dissect an ape and learn each of the bones from it by carefully removing the flesh. For this, you must choose apes which most resemble man. These are apes which do not have prominent jaws or large canine teeth. In these apes which also walk and run on two legs, you will also find the other parts as in man. Those apes, however, which are like the dog headed baboons have larger muscles and large canine teeth. They have difficulty in standing upright on two legs, let alone walking or running.

(*On Anatomical Procedures* Book 1, chapter 2)

Though Galen assumed sensibly, and for most purposes correctly, that the anatomy of human beings and other mammals were closely similar, he did on occasions make some mistakes about human anatomy. Nevertheless because of his dissections Galen acquired a great deal of accurate and valuable information about anatomy.

Galen and physiology

Galen's investigations did not end with anatomy. He was also interested in physiology. He developed a far-reaching, if incorrect, theory of the movement of the blood. He probably also realised that there was a circulation of the blood through the lungs. The working of the nervous system was another of Galen's interests and he conducted a number of experiments on the spinal cords of pigs:

Your dissection of the spinal marrow should be made in the following manner. Provide yourself with a large strong knife . . . The animal which you vivisect should not be old—so that it will be easy for you to cut through the vertebrae [the bones of the spine] . . . Now assume that you have already done what is here described, so that the spinal marrow lies exposed . . . If you wish to paralyse all the parts of the body below this section and stop any movement . . . then sever the spinal marrow with a cut running completely through so that no parts remain joined together . . . [If you cut the spinal marrow near] to the thoracic vertebrae, then the first thing that happens is that you see the animal's respiration and voice have been damaged . . . if you cut through . . . behind the fifth vertebrae of the head . . . then both arms are paralysed.

(*On Anatomical Procedures* Book 9, chapter 13)

The influence of Galen

Galen's ideas had enormous influence, lasting for over 1200 years. During his lifetime Galen wrote a great number of books, in which he produced a complete system of medicine. The system included not only Galen's own observations, but also the ideas of Hippocrates, Erasistratus, Herophilus and other Greek physicians. Galen's books provided doctors with a mass of detailed and well organised information. Galen's descriptions of anatomy and physiology were all influenced by the theory that all organs in the body had been produced by a 'Creator' for some definite purpose. Such ideas made a special appeal in later times to both Christian and Muslim churches. This might help to explain why so many of Galen's works survived the following centuries, and continued to have an important influence on doctors during the middle ages.

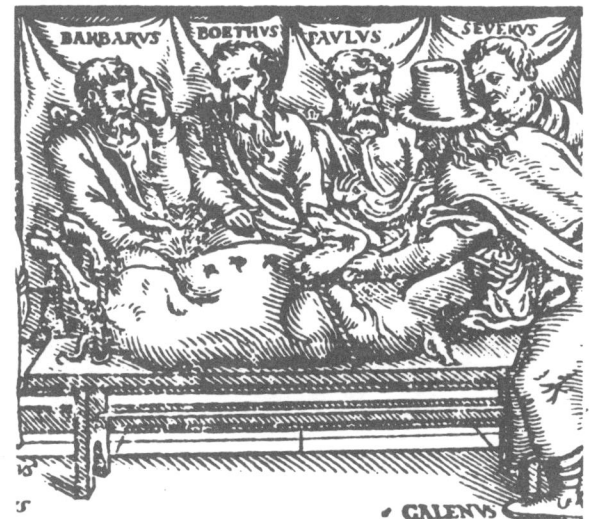

Glossary

acute   a word used to describe an illness which develops quickly to a crisis point, after which the patient either dies or recovers

aedile   a Roman government official responsible for repairing public buildings, sewers, streets, aqueducts, etc. They had power to fine people causing damage

amphora   a storage jar

anise   the oily, scented seed of a plant which was useful in stomach medicines

aqueduct   a channel for carrying water which was usually supported on stone arches (like a bridge)

balm   thick golden coloured oil produced by the balsam tree and used to help heal wounds and stop infection

bile   a brownish-yellow, bitter liquid (produced by the liver) which helps to digest food. There is in fact only yellow bile. Black bile was probably stale blood

booty   stolen goods gained in war

caldarium   the hot room in the baths

canopic jar   a stone or clay jar produced in the Egyptian town of Canopus used for holding the internal organs of embalmed bodies

cassia   a plant whose roots produce a fragrant and highly scented perfume

cautery   a heated metal instrument or a drug which is placed on an open wound to burn it and so help it heal

censor   a Roman government official responsible for collecting taxes and arranging contracts for the repair of public buildings, aqueducts, sewers etc.

ceramic   made of clay

cholera   a serious disease caught from contaminated food or water. It causes violent vomiting and diarrhoea and can result in death from dehydration—loss of water from the body

cistern   water tank

clinical   at the patient's sickbed

code   a set of rules

colocynth   the seeds or pulp of sour yellow fruit which, when eaten, help to clear out the bowels

commissioner   a person given the power to carry out certain duties

consuls   the two chief Roman government officials

cult   system of religious worship

cumin   the seeds of a small plant which produce oil useful as a stomach medicine

decoction   a liquid produced by boiling something down to extract the essence

diagnose   to identify a disease by means of a patient's symptoms

diaphragm   a band of muscle which separates the chest and the abdomen

dysentery   severe diarrhoea caused by an infection in the bowels

embalmer   the person who treats a dead body with salt, oil and spices in order to preserve it from decay

extracted   taken out, removed

figs   fruits of the fig tree—when they are eaten they help to clear out the bowels; syrup of figs is still taken today

flint   a very hard grey stone

frankincense   scented white gum obtained from the bark of the olibanum tree

frescoes   paintings done on plastered walls

garlic   the bulb of a small plant which has a taste similar to an onion

hellebore   a plant also known as 'Christmas rose'—its roots were used as a medicine to clear out the bowels: in fact they were poisonous

humour   liquid, fluid

ibex   a wild goat with reddish brown hair

ingenious   clever

innate   inborn, natural

lore   beliefs, traditions, ideas

eches   blood sucking worms

vid   a bluish, leaden colour

hortar   a basin in which herbs etc. were pounded with a pestle

hucus   slimy liquid usually found in the nose

hyrrh   yellow gum produced by the bark of a small tree. The gum contains a tiny amount of antiseptic and is used as a stomach medicine or to embalm bodies

atron   a kind of salt

omadic   wandering from place to place

chre   earth containing iron oxide which varies in colour from pale yellow to deep red

racle   the advice of a god spoken or interpreted through a priestess or priest

re   rock containing some kind of metal

rgan   a part of a human or animal body such as the lungs, heart, etc.

apyrus   a kind of paper made from thin strips of papyrus reed

erch   a spiny freshwater fish

estle   a club-shaped tool used for pounding herbs and other substances in a mortar (bowl)

phlegm   a thick slimy fluid usually produced in the throat. It was regarded as one of the four humours (cold and moist)

polyps   small lumps or swellings

praetor   a Roman government official who acted as a judge in the law courts

pus   thick yellow liquid produced in an infected wound

pustule   a pimple

quartz   hard white crystals found in rocks

ro   an Egyptian unit of measurement equal to about one teaspoonful

senna   the leaves of a small plant which when ground up and eaten help to clear out the bowels. Senna pods or pills made from senna are still used today

spices   strongly scented seeds, leaves or roots of plants often used to help preserve dead bodies

spleen   an internal organ of the body found near the stomach

squills   the bulb of a lily plant

stadium (plural: stadia)   a Greek measurement of length equal to $606\frac{3}{4}$ feet, or about 184 metres. Because in Greece foot races were 606 (Greek) feet long the word stadium came to describe the place where the race was run

stibium   burnt antimony (a kind of metal substance) which can be used either as a poison or to clear out the bowels

technology   science used for practical purposes

tepidarium   the warm room in the baths

terracotta   made of baked clay

tumour   a swelling or lump

typhoid   a serious disease caught from contaminated food or water. It causes high fever and ulcers in the intestines. Patients often die from internal bleeding

verjuice   the acid liquid from sour grapes or crab apples

vertebrae   the small bones which make up the back bone (or spine)

virulent   poisonous

vizier   a chief minister or adviser

vomiting   being sick

votive   offered in thanksgiving

wehedu   something which caused pus to form

Acknowledgements

The authors and publishers are grateful to the following for permission to reproduce copyright material:

Photographs and illustrations

page 4   *a prehistoric case of clubfoot, the femur of a prehistoric man*, Trustees of the British Museum (Natural History);

page 5   *cave painting from southern France*, Mansell Collection; *prehistoric skull, etc.*, Anthropological Institute, Florence;

page 6   *an Aboriginal shelter*, Popperfoto;

page 7   *a sacred churinga stone*, Australian Information Service;

page 8   *Aborigine Emu dancers, bullroarer, landscape*, Australian Information Service;

page 9   *a Medicine Man in the Northern Territory*, Australian Information Service;

page 10   *a Medicine Man*, Herald & Weekly Times, Melbourne (fig. C p. 141 from *Wanderings in Wild Australia*, Sir Baldwin Spencer);

page 11   *a charm made from a human hand*, National Museum of Australia; *redseed charm*, Trustees of the Australian Museum, College Street, Sydney;

page 13   *the god Khum*, Mansell Collection; *the gods Osiris and Isis*, Historical Picture Service;

page 14   *funeral inscription to Irj*, Trustees of the British Museum;

page 15   *Sekhmet, the war goddess*, Mansell Collection;

page 16   *a column from Papyrus Edwin Smith*, Trustees of the British Museum;

page 17   *a mummy found at Thebes*, Trustees of the British Museum; *tomb painting showing a soul returning to the body*, Historical Picture Service;

page 19   *stone carving from the temple of Kom Ombo*, by courtesy of the Wellcome Trustees;

page 20   *a tomb painting*, Trustees of the British Museum; *lady vomiting at a banquet, jewelled charm*, Mansell Collection;

page 22   *Syrian prince, Nebamon*, Trustees of the British Museum;

page 23   *an early Greek jug*, Trustees of the British Museum;

page 24   *Greek gold coin*, Hirmer Fotoarchiv, München;

page 25   *statue of Asclepios*, Mansell Collection;

page 26   *fifth century frieze showing Asclepios healing*, Mansell Collection;

page 27   *a Greek ship*, Clarendon Press, Oxford (from *A History of Technology*, Vol II, Fig. 99, p. 130); *plate of baked clay*, Abelard-Schuman Limited;

page 28   *bust of Hippocrates*, Mansell Collection;

page 29   *tombstone of Jason*, Mansell Collection;

page 31   *bronze bleeding cup*, Trustees of the British Museum;

page 32   *running man*, Trustees of the British Museum;

page 33   *Greek women taking a shower bath*, Clarendon Press, Oxford (from *A History of Technology*, Vol II, Fig. 610, p. 667);

page 34   *Hippocrates studying a patient's urine*, Instituto Serono, Rome;

page 35   *treatment for displaced vertebrae*, Biblioteca Medicea Laurenziana, photograph by G. Pineider; *surgical instruments*, Instituto Serono, Rome;

page 36   *Triple Arch of the Emperor Constantine*, Mansell Collection;

page 37   *bridge across the Tagus*, Radio Times Hulton Picture Library;

page 38   *Roman marble inscription*, Mansell Collection;

page 39   *reconstruction of the Queen's bathroom at Knossos*, Agathon Press, U.S.A.

page 42   *Pont du Gard aqueduct, Nimes*, Spectrum Colour Library;

page 46   *plan of Bath House at Vindolanda*, Mr Robin Birley, The Vindolanda Trust, Bardon Mill, Hexham, Northumberland; *public latrines at Housesteads*, Crown Copyright, reproduced with the permission of the Controller of Her Majesty's Stationery Office;

page 47   *outlet into the Tiber of the 'Cloaca Maxima'*, Trustees of the British Museum; *public latrines at Leptis Magna*, Ms G. Farnell;

page 49   *model reconstruction of tenement block*, Mansell Collection;

page 50   *Roman surgical and midwifery instruments*, Mansell Collection;

page 51   *portrait of Galen*, Civica Raccolta Stampe A. Berterelli-Milano;

page 52   *title page from Galen, and detail*, by courtesy of the Wellcome Trustees.

Extracts

Adapted from the following translations:

page 14   A. H. Gardiner in *The Legacy of Egypt*, p. 77 ed. S. R. K. Glanville, OUP 1942;

page 15   Remedies from the Papyrus Ebers, Papyrus Edwin Smith and Papyrus Berlin based on translations by B. Ebbell, *The Papyrus Ebers: The Greatest Egyptian Medical Document*, Copenhagen 1939; J. Breasted, *Edwin Smith Surgical Papyrus*, University of Chicago Press, 1930; A. Erman, *Zauberspruche fur mutter und kind aus dem Papyrus 3027 der Berliner Museum*, Berlin 1901;

Herodotus references are adapted from D. D. Godley *Loeb classics*, Heinemann 1921;

Hippocrates extracts adapted from W. H. S. Jones, *Loeb classics*, Heinemann 1923;

page 27   extract from *An Illustrated history of science* by F. Sherwood Taylor, pp 1-2, Heinemann 1955;

page 35   extract from *Greek Medicine* by E. D. Philips, Thames & Hudson, p. 14, 1975;

Thucydides extracts from Rex Warner's translation of *History of the Peloponnesian War*, Book 2, Penguin Books, 1954;

Extracts from Pliny, *Natural History* and Strabo, *Geography* adapted from translations by W. H. S. Jones, Heinemann 1923.

The authors and publishers have made every effort to trace copyright owners of material used in this book. In cases where they have been unsuccessful they apologise for any accidental infringement of copyright.